Praise for the Second
101 Questions & Answers about

"This book is absolutely superb, a great resource for both patients as well as primary-care providers (including MDs, NPs, PAs, etc.). A real tour de force! It should be a must for all patients with hypertension who want to be educated about their condition."

— **Phyllis August, MD, MPH**
Ralph A. Baer Professor of Research in Medicine
and Director, Hypertension Center
Weill Cornell Medical Center/New York-Presbyterian Hospital, New York, NY

"After reviewing the text of this book, it is clear that it is timely and written such that everyone from the nonprofessional to physicians can garner important pearls for understanding the disease. This is not surprising since the first edition of this book, published in 2001, was coedited by two giants in the field, the late great Ray W. Gifford, Jr., and the alive and well William Manger.

This latest update, however, continues to improve with readability and flow that is effortless, with every page providing a pearl. Dr. Norman M. Kaplan has teamed up with Dr. Manger for the latest edition, which is better than the previous one, if that is possible. The book answers all the questions any patient could ask and provides updated facts to back up all major statements. A must read for the more than 72 million people who suffer from hypertension or those who have loved ones with the disease. A great effort from great physicians."

— **George Bakris, MD**
Professor of Medicine and Director, Hypertensive Diseases Unit
The University of Chicago Prizker School of Medicine

"The book provides a comprehensive and informative look at blood pressure and hypertension. Written for the patient but informative for the expert, it is written in an easily understood format. It can be used as a reference for the particular question you might have or read in its entirety from cover-to-cover to gain a comprehensive understanding of hypertension. "

— **Jan Basile, MD**
Former Chief, Primary Care Service Line, Ralph H. Johnson VAMC
Professor of Medicine, Medical University of South Carolina, Charleston, SC

"Dr. Manger has done it again. The second edition of his book *100 Questions and Answers about Hypertension* has been thoroughly and

skillfully updated and serves as a very valuable resource for anyone interested in any and all aspects of hypertension. ... I enthusiastically recommend it for patients, potential patients, families of patients, and also for health-care providers who care for patients with hypertension."
— **Henry R. Black, MD, MACP,** Clinical Professor of Internal Medicine, Center for the Prevention of Cardiovascular Disease Emeritus President, American Society of Hypertension, 2008–1010

"I have read your book and it is indeed superb! The book provides highly reliable information in an understandable form on virtually all aspects of blood pressure and hypertension. The book is both useful to read in its entirety and valuable in addressing answers to key questions as they arise. I will recommend it for my patients as an essential resource in their care."
— **Robert M. Carey, MD, MACP**
David A. Harrison III Distinguished Professor of Medicine, Dean, Emeritus, and University Professor Division of Endocrinology and Metabolism, University of Virginia Health System, Charlottesville, VA

"The question-and-answer approach is used very effectively as an educational tool to convey the most important clinical messages regarding hypertension. The book is recommended for both hypertensive patients and the general public."
— **Aram V. Chobanian, MD**
President Emeritus, Boston University Dean and Provost Emeritus Boston University School of Medicine

"Dr. William Manger has updated his and the late Dr. Ray Gifford's earlier volume with highly regarded colleagues Dr. Norman Kaplan and Edward Roccella. Dr. Gifford was 'the' physician's physician to all seeking his advice about hypertensive diseases. These four authorities clearly deal with extremely important and highly relevant clinical questions that provide insightful and very meaningful answers to physicians and patients alike."
— **Edward D. Frohlich, MD, MACP, FACC**
Alton Ochsner Distinguished Scientist, Ochsner Clinic Foundation, New Orleans, LA Former Editor-in-Chief, American Heart Association's journal *Hypertension*

"The book is an excellent resource for primary-care or family physicians and nurse practitioners, as well as for hypertensive patients who seek reliable background information."
— **Haralambos P. Gavras, MD, and Irene Gavras, MD**
Professors of Medicine, Boston University School of Medicine, Boston, MA

"There is nothing better to inform the public about hypertension."

— Francis J. Haddy, MD, PhD
Emeritus Professor and Chair of Physiology at the University of Oklahoma,
Michigan State University, and the Uniformed Services University,
Current Member of the Graduate Faculty Department of Physiology and
Bioengineering, Mayo Clinic College of Medicine

"This book is a definitive and useful resource for patients with hypertension. Laypeople will find the answers to each of the 101 questions readable, brief, and clear. The text is thorough and accessible. Great teachers manage to simplify the complex, and the authors have admirably succeeded in doing so here."

— Jules Manger, MD
Retired emergency physician, past director emergency department
and co-director trauma service, Concord Hospital, Concord, NH
Founding partner and past president, Concord Emergency Medical Associates
Past director, emergency medical services for central NH
Former adjunct teaching staff, Dartmouth Medical School

"101 Questions translates the medical knowledge of hypertension into understandable bytes of information. I recommend it."

— Samuel J. Mann, MD
Professor of Clinical Medicine, Division of Nephrology and Hypertension
New York-Presbyterian Hospital/Weill Cornell Medical Center

"Drs. Manger, Kaplan, and Roccella have done an excellent job of posing and answering many of the questions that people have about high blood pressure, what it is, what it does, and what you can do about it. They are to be congratulated for clarifying and correcting many of the myths and misconceptions about this disease."

— Marvin M. Moser, MD
Clinical Professor of Medicine, Yale School of Medicine
Emeritus Editor, Journal of Clinical Hypertension

"This book is great for doctors and medical students!"

— Sir Stanley W. Peart, MD, London, England

"The 101 questions and answers prepared by top experts on hypertension represent an excellent tool to achieve a healthy lifestyle and successfully manage high blood pressure."

— Alberto Zanchetti, MD
Emeritus Professor of Medicine, University of Milan
Past-President, International Society of Hypertension
Past-President, European Society of Hypertension

Ordering
Trade bookstores in the U.S. and Canada please contact:

Publishers Group West
1700 Fourth Street, Berkeley CA 94710
Phone: (800) 788-3123   Fax: (800) 351-5073

Hunter House books are available at bulk discounts for textbook course
adoptions; to qualifying community, health-care, and government
organizations; and for special promotions and fund-raising.
For details please contact:

Special Sales Department
Hunter House Inc., PO Box 2914, Alameda CA 94501-0914
Phone: (510) 865-5282   Fax: (510) 865-4295
E-mail: ordering@hunterhouse.com

Individuals can order our books from most bookstores,
by calling **(800) 266-5592**, or from our website at
www.hunterhouse.com

101 Questions & Answers about Hypertension

~ SECOND EDITION ~

William M. Manger, MD, PhD
Norman M. Kaplan, MD

with

Ray W. Gifford, Jr., MD
and Edward J. Roccella, PhD, MPH

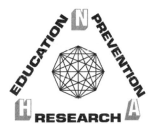

NATIONAL HYPERTENSION ASSOCIATION

PUBLISHERS

Hunter House Inc., Publishers
PO Box 2914
Alameda CA 94501-0914

Library of Congress Cataloging-in-Publication Data
101 questions and answers about hypertension /
William M. Manger... [et al.]. — 2nd ed.
p. cm.
Rev. ed. of: 100 questions and answers about hypertension / by William M.
Manger and Ray W. Gifford, Jr. c2001.
ISBN 978-0-89793-571-5 (pbk.)
1. Hypertension — Miscellanea. 2. Hypertension — Popular works.
I. Manger, William Muir, 1920– II. Manger, William Muir, 1920– 100 questions
and answers about hypertension. III. Title: One hundred and
one questions and answers about hypertension. IV. Title: One hundred
one questions and answers about hypertension.
RC685.H8M277 2011
616.1'32 — dc23   2011014362

Project Credits

Cover Design: Brian Dittmar Graphics   Intern: Erica M. Lee
Book Production: John McKercher   Publicity and Marketing: Sean Harvey
Copy Editor: Amy Bauman   Order Fulfillment: Washul Lakdhon
Proofreader: John David Marion   Administrator: Theresa Nelson
Indexer: Candace Hyatt   Computer Support: Peter Eichelberger
Managing Editor: Alexandra Mummery   Acquisitions Assistant: Elizabeth Kracht
Senior Marketing Associate: Reina Santana
Rights Coordinator: Candace Groskreutz
Customer Service Manager: Christina Sverdrup
Publisher: Kiran S. Rana

Printed and bound by Bang Printing, Brainerd, Minnesota
Manufactured in the United States of America

....   9 8 7 6 5 4 3 2 1   Second Edition   11 12 13 14 15   ....

— Contents

— Foreword

An important need exists for increasing public and patient awareness and knowledge regarding high blood pressure, or hypertension. An illness whose prevalence continues to increase, hypertension currently afflicts more than 72 million adults here in the United States. Blood pressure increases steadily with age. More than 60 percent of men and women over the age of sixty-five have elevated levels of blood pressure, and if one lives long enough, the risk of developing hypertension in one's lifetime is greater than 90 percent. At any age, the higher the blood pressure, the greater the risk for cardiovascular diseases including heart attacks, heart failure, angina, stroke, and kidney diseases. High blood pressure is a major cause of death and disability and ranks in importance with abnormal blood cholesterol levels and smoking as a major risk factor for cardiovascular diseases.

Even modest increases in blood pressure can be detrimental to the cardiovascular system, whereas small reductions of blood pressure in the population, particularly in those considered to be "prehypertensive," can have significant positive benefits. Lifestyle approaches to lower blood pressure, such as weight reduction, increased physical activity, and dietary changes that favor a reduction in salt or sodium chloride and an increased intake of foods that are high in potassium, grains, fruits, vegetables, and nonfat dairy products should be promoted for the population as a whole. Obesity is not only a cause of hypertension, but it also contributes to abnormal blood fats and diabetes. Unfortunately, the prevalence of obesity has increased significantly during the past quarter century and has contributed greatly to the rise in prevalence of hypertension observed during this period.

Advances in drug therapy during the past fifty years have had a major impact on the ability to control hypertension. The capability now exists to normalize blood pressure in most hypertensive individuals. In addition, many clinical studies have confirmed the major benefits of blood pressure lowering in reducing the incidence of serious cardiovascular complications. Despite these well-known benefits, control of hypertension, even in affluent countries such as ours, remains inadequate. Many factors may be responsible for the poor control. The most important of these are inadequate attention of physicians to management of elevated blood pressure, failure of patients to adhere to prescribed therapy on a long-term basis, and issues related to access to and cost of treatment.

Hypertension is a chronic disease that usually requires long-term therapy. In his or her lifetime, the typical hypertensive patient is likely to receive many different medications that may vary in their mechanism of action and have different beneficial or adverse effects. The patients also may be asked to make major lifestyle changes and may elect to use "alternative" therapy to manage the hypertension. The diverse nature of these therapies and of the various contributing causes of hypertension have created an environment that has bred many misconceptions and myths about the disease. Therefore, the need is great for authoritative sources of information on hypertension to guide patients.

Although several quality publications exist for public and patient education on hypertension and cardiovascular diseases, none has utilized so effectively the question/answer approach that has been provided in this book by Drs. Manger, Kaplan, and Roccella, all of whom are leaders in the field of hypertension. They answer the most commonly asked questions on hypertension in a clear and comprehensive manner and cover many important aspects of the problem, including the prevention of hypertension and the need to focus on the growing prevalence of obesity in youth. The book represents a valuable addition to the field, and I would recommend it both for patients and for others interested in knowing more about the disease. It also has value as an educational tool for health-care providers who deal frequently with hypertensive patients.

— Aram V. Chobanian, MD
Emeritus Dean and Provost, Boston University School of Medicine
Emeritus President, Boston University, Boston, Massachusetts

Important Note

The material in this book is intended to provide a review of information regarding hypertension. It is an educational book for lay and paramedical personnel; people who have or suspect they might have hypertension or prehypertension should always consult a doctor regarding treatment of these conditions. Every effort has been made to provide accurate and dependable information. The contents of this book have been compiled through professional research and in consultation with medical and mental-health professionals. However, health-care professionals have differing opinions, and advances in medical and scientific research are made very quickly, so some of the information presented in this book may become outdated.

Therefore, the publisher, authors, and editors, as well as the professionals quoted in the book, cannot be held responsible for any error, omission, or dated material. The authors and publisher assume no responsibility for any outcome of applying the information in this book in a program of self-care or under the care of a licensed practitioner. If you have questions concerning hypertension or about the application of the information described in this book, consult a qualified health-care professional.

— Acknowledgments

I feel compelled to praise those involved in the preparation of this timely book.

The late Ray W. Gifford, Jr., was a coauthor of the first edition of *100 Questions and Answers about Hypertension*, which was published in 2001. Ray, who served as past chairman of the Department of Nephrology and Hypertension at the Cleveland Clinic, was regarded by his peers as one of the most knowledgeable and talented clinical hypertension experts on the planet.

Dr. Norman M. Kaplan kindly agreed to help update this second edition of *100 Questions and Answers about Hypertension*. No one is more qualified to step in for Dr. Gifford. Dr. Kaplan has enormous expertise in clinical hypertension. His textbook *Clinical Hypertension*, which he periodically updates, continues to be the premier guide for physicians involved in diagnosing and managing patients with hypertension.

Dr. Edward Roccella has had enormous experience in the field of hypertension, and he combined his talent with that of Dr. Claude Lenfant (former director of the National Heart, Lung, and Blood Institute) to effectively lead the National High Blood Pressure Education Program for many years at the National Institutes of Health. His expertise has very significantly improved the context of this book.

This second edition of *100 Questions and Answers about Hypertension* was written for the public, but paramedical personnel and physicians should also find it very helpful for their patients who have hypertension.

We wish to express deep gratitude for excellent comments and constructive suggestions by many of the most distinguished hypertension experts in the nation:

Phyllis August, MD
George L. Bakris, MD
Jan Basile, MD
Henry R. Black, MD
Robert M. Carey, MD
Aram V. Chobanian, MD
Edward D. Frohlich, MD
Haralambos P. Gavras, MD
Irene Gavras, MD
Francis J. Haddy, MD, PhD
Jules N. Manger, MD
Samuel J. Mann, MD
Marvin M. Moser, MD
Sir Stanley W. Peart, MD
Alberto Zanchetti, MD

We also wish to express special gratitude to Alla Krayko for outstanding secretarial assistance and to Ruth Johnston and Richard Ruge for their exceptional help in proofreading.

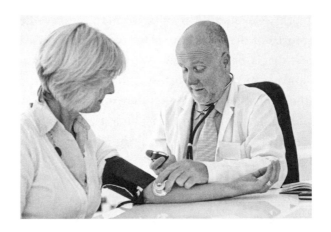

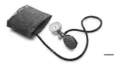

1 What Is Blood Pressure?

Blood pressure (BP) is the force exerted by the blood on the walls of the arteries. The pressure depends on the amount of blood pumped by the heart plus the resistance the blood meets, which is caused mainly by the degree of constriction of the smallest arteries called *arterioles*. These arterioles have smooth muscle in their walls that can contract or relax, thereby altering the caliber (lumen, or size) of the vessels. Constriction of these vessels and increasing resistance to flow will raise pressure — the effect has been likened to reducing the opening at a hose's nozzle to impede the flow of water and thus elevating the pressure of water in the hose. Pressure in the

> Blood pressure is the pressure exerted by the blood on the walls of the arteries.

hose can also be increased by increasing the amount of water flowing from the faucet; this effect is analogous to the increased blood flow that ensues when the force with which the heart beats and/or the heart rate is augmented.

BP varies considerably during the day, depending on the demands of the body. For example, BP will increase markedly during exercise, when muscles require a greater supply of oxygen and nutrition. This elevated BP results from an increased rate and pumping force of the heart; the arterioles in the muscles actually dilate — that is, become larger — to permit an increased blood supply. Similarly, anxiety during the "fight-or-flight" response can activate the sympathetic nervous system and cause the liberation of epinephrine and similar hormones; as a result, the heart speeds up and pumps out more blood even as the arterioles become constricted, thereby increasing BP.

During sleep, inactivity reduces the demand for oxygen. The rate and pumping force of the heart therefore decrease and the arterioles relax and dilate. As a result, the BP decreases. Normally, pressure is lowest at night and highest in the morning when arousal activates the sympathetic nervous system. Although BP remains primarily under the control of the nervous system, a variety of substances and hormones released from the kidneys, heart, adrenal glands, and the lining of the blood vessels play an important role in altering the caliber of the arterioles and can elevate or lower blood pressure in response to a variety of stressful conditions. Under normal circumstances, the arterioles are relatively relaxed and dilated, and the BP remains in a normal range.

2 What Are Systolic, Diastolic, and Pulse Pressures?

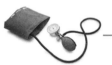

Blood pressure (BP) is the force that blood exerts on the walls of the arteries as a result of the pumping force of the heart. It is determined by the amount of blood that the heart pumps every beat as well as by the resistance that the blood meets in the smaller blood vessels called *arterioles*. Anything that tends to constrict or narrow the arterioles will raise BP; conversely, anything that relaxes them will lower BP. An increase in the amount of blood that is pumped by the heart will not necessarily increase BP if the arterioles dilate to lessen the resistance that the blood meets.

Systolic BP is the pressure generated by each beat of the heart. It is so named because each beat or contraction of the heart is known as a "systole." *Diastolic BP* is the pressure between heartbeats, when the heart is not contracting; this event is known as "diastole." Systolic BP is always higher than diastolic BP because it is generated by the force of the heartbeat. BP is usually expressed as systolic BP over diastolic BP in millimeters of mercury (for example, 130/80 mm Hg*). Pulse pressure is the difference between systolic and diastolic

> Pulse pressure is the difference between systolic and diastolic blood pressure.

BPs. For example, when the systolic pressure is 130 mm Hg and the diastolic pressure is 80 mm Hg (130/80), the pulse pressure is 50 (130 − 80 = 50). Significant elevation of any of these pressures increases the risk of heart disease, stroke, and kidney disease.

3 How Is Blood Pressure Measured?

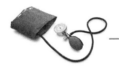

In the doctor's office, blood pressure (BP) is usually measured with a stethoscope and a sphygmomanometer. The latter instrument contains a glass tube in which the height of a mercury column indicates the pressure. Some instruments have a gauge, and others have a digital readout to measure BP. Measuring BP is quite simple, painless, and quick.

> In the doctor's office, blood pressure is usually measured with a stethoscope and a sphygmomanometer.

The sphygmomanometer consists of a cloth cuff containing an inflatable rubber bag, which is connected by a rubber tube to a device such as a reservoir of mercury or a spring gauge (see Figure 1 on the next page). The cuff is wrapped around the patient's upper arm, with the lower edge remaining approximately one inch above the arm crease. Repeatedly squeezing a rubber bulb pumps air through another tube into the rubber bag. The pressure in the bag, which is the same as that elevating the column of mercury,

---

* Hg is the chemical symbol for mercury.

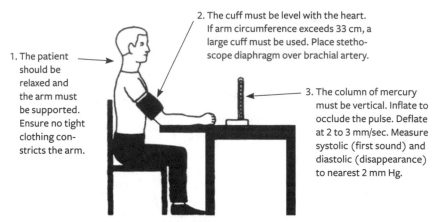

1. The patient should be relaxed and the arm must be supported. Ensure no tight clothing constricts the arm.

2. The cuff must be level with the heart. If arm circumference exceeds 33 cm, a large cuff must be used. Place stethoscope diaphragm over brachial artery.

3. The column of mercury must be vertical. Inflate to occlude the pulse. Deflate at 2 to 3 mm/sec. Measure systolic (first sound) and diastolic (disappearance) to nearest 2 mm Hg.

Figure 1. Technique of blood pressure measurement recommended by the British Hypertension Society (Source: "Blood Pressure Measurement: Techniques Recommended by the British Hypertension Society." *Journal of Hypertension* 3 (1985): 293–95.)

increases until it temporarily stops the flow of blood in the arm. At this point, the listening device of a stethoscope is placed over the inner side of the elbow crease, just below the cuff. When blood flow is stopped, no heart sound is heard with the stethoscope. Air is then gradually released through a valve in the rubber bulb, which slowly reduces the pressure in the bag; the mercury column will fall at the same time. The moment at which the first thumping sound is heard through the stethoscope, the level of the mercury column in millimeters is recorded as the systolic pressure; it indicates the pressure when the heart is contracting and the blood begins to flow through the arm. As the pressure in the bag continues to fall, the thumping sounds (which are due to spurts of blood with each heart contraction) will no longer be heard. This point is recorded in millimeters of mercury as the diastolic pressure (see Figure 2).

BP is recorded as systolic BP over diastolic BP and is recorded with two numbers as follows:

$$\frac{\text{systolic}}{\text{diastolic}} \text{ mm Hg (millimeters of mercury)}$$

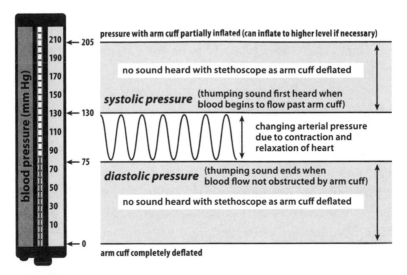

pressure with arm cuff partially inflated (can inflate to higher level if necessary)

no sound heard with stethoscope as arm cuff deflated

systolic pressure (thumping sound first heard when blood begins to flow past arm cuff)

changing arterial pressure due to contraction and relaxation of heart

diastolic pressure (thumping sound ends when blood flow not obstructed by arm cuff)

no sound heard with stethoscope as arm cuff deflated

arm cuff completely deflated

blood pressure (mm Hg)

Figure 2. Blood pressure measurement in arm with sphygmomanometer and stethoscope

Normal systolic pressures for adults more than eighteen years old usually range from 100 to 120 mm Hg and diastolic pressures from 60 to 80 mm Hg. Systolic pressures of 120 to 139 mm Hg and diastolic pressures of 80 to 89 mm Hg, formerly considered high normal, are now considered elevated and are called prehypertensive. In general, people with relatively low systolic and diastolic pressures are less likely to develop strokes, heart disease, or kidney disease (see Figure 2).

Another device for measuring BP is the aneroid sphygmomanometer, which incorporates a gauge that indicates blood pressure by measuring the tension of a spring instead of the height of a mercury column; however, a stethoscope is required. Electronic sphygmomanometers with a digital display of the BP and pulse rate are especially convenient because they do not require a stethoscope. We recommend the use of such instruments with an arm cuff. Digital finger and wrist cuffs are usually less accurate. Electronic sphygmomanometers have an especially desirable feature — the rubber bag in the cuff can be automatically inflated and deflated by simply pressing a button. (The Omron HEM-704C,

Omron 705CP and X, and Sunbeam 7650 self-inflating sphygmo-manometers have been reported to be quite accurate and simple for the patient to use at home.)

Increasingly, BP determined both in the doctor's office and at home is being measured with electronic devices that sense pulsation in the artery. Here the balloon in the cuff on the arm is automatically filled with air to a level that temporarily stops blood circulation in the arm, at which point the recorder detects no pulsations. As the pressure in the balloon is lowered, circulation resumes and the first pulsation is recorded as the systolic BP. When the cuff pressure no longer impedes blood flow in the artery beneath the cuff, the pulsations disappear and at this point the device records the diastolic BP.

BP will usually be similar in both arms. No matter which arm is used, BP should be determined when the patient is in the seated position, because the risks of elevated BP have been determined based on studies of BPs taken from seated patients. Additional information may be obtained by measuring BP in the recumbent and standing positions, as these data may help establish whether BP is normal in these positions and whether treatment effectively controls BP in all positions.

Many home devices include a cuff/balloon that is too small for obese or highly muscular people. If the cuff/balloon does not go easily around the upper arm, a wider and longer cuff/balloon should be used. Some devices include a larger, or thigh, cuff/balloon. If a particular device does not include this additional piece, one can be ordered from the manufacturer. Small cuffs are available for children.

It is especially important that a person remain seated with their back supported and rest in a quiet environment for at least five minutes before BP measurements are taken. Cigarette smoking, consumption of drinks containing caffeine, and exercise should be avoided for about one hour before the BP is measured. Crossing the legs and even just talking can elevate BP. It is also important that the arm cuff be at the level of the heart (that is, the level of the breast bone) and that the proper size cuff is used, which depends on the size of the arm.

Be prepared for rather marked differences between readings even when taken a few minutes apart. BP varies even under stable conditions and more so with physical activity, smoking, the consumption of coffee or tea, and emotional distress. You will soon become accustomed to such normal variability.

You can easily determine to what degree various activities affect your blood pressure. Take a series of readings before and then twenty minutes after a cup of strong coffee or after an argument with your spouse over who will take out the trash. If you find on more than one reading that your BP goes up more than 10 mm Hg after any such activity, try to avoid that activity (e.g., drink fewer cups of coffee). There is no need to limit normal activity that usually raises BP only slightly.

Take your home device to the doctor's office and have the nurse take your pressure with the office device on one arm at the same time as you take a reading on the other arm. If the simultaneously taken BP readings differ by more than 10 mm Hg, change arms with the nurse to see if one arm is consistently higher than the other. If so, use the arm with the higher reading for taking measurements at home. This is a good way to determine if your home device is functioning properly.

4 What Is Normal Blood Pressure?

For many years, 140/90 mm Hg was considered the dividing line between normal and high blood pressure (BP), or at least it was widely accepted as the upper limit for which life insurance would be issued. Observational studies have since shown conclusively that risk begins with any systolic BP above 115 mm Hg and with any diastolic BP above 75 mm Hg. Optimal BP is 120/80 or less, prehypertension is 120–139 systolic or 80–89 diastolic.

Recognizing the increased cardiovascular risk when the BP is above "normal," 120/80 mm Hg, but not at or above 140/90 mm Hg, defined as "hypertensive," the *Seventh Report of the Joint National Committee on Prevention, Detection, Evaluation, and Treatment of High Blood Pressure* (*JNC7*), published in 2003, recommends that pressures in this intermediate range be defined as "prehypertensive." *JNC7* did not recommend that drug therapy should be given to people with prehypertension but rather that these patients focus on more intensive attempts to change unhealthy lifestyles such as smoking, excessive weight, and lack of physical activity. Recommendations from British and European expert committees have not yet incorporated this definition, but all agree that such people should have their BP checked more frequently and improve their health habits.

> *Optimal blood pressure is 120/80 mm Hg or less, normal blood pressure is less than 130/80 mm Hg, and high-normal pressure is 130–139/85–89 mm Hg.*

It should be realized that one determination of BP may not be representative of the usual BP — particularly if the reading is high or low. For this reason, most physicians do not initiate treatment on the basis of a single elevated BP reading unless it is extremely high or unless the patient already has some evidence of "target organ disease" (such as damage to the heart, brain, kidneys, or eyes) or additional risk factors. Such risk factors may include elevated "bad" cholesterol (low-density lipoprotein [LDL] cholesterol) or triglyceride levels in the blood, cigarette smoking, diabetes mellitus, a sedentary lifestyle, and a family history of premature heart attack or stroke in a parent or sibling.

5 Are the Blood Pressure Machines in Pharmacies, Shopping Malls, Airports, and Other Public Places Accurate?

The blood pressure (BP) machines found in public places may be accurate if they are properly calibrated when they are first installed and are also checked and recalibrated frequently (especially if they are used often). Unless you know a particular device is serviced regularly, it is hardly worth the effort to use it because of the aggravation that an erroneous reading may produce. In addition, checking your BP after paying a large grocery bill at the supermarket may not be the best time to determine your usual BP reading!

> The blood pressure machines found in public places may be accurate if they are properly calibrated and are also checked and recalibrated frequently.

To ensure the most accurate BP recordings, it is important to remember that the individual should be seated and at rest for at least five minutes before the pressure is measured (see Question 3). If others are waiting to use the sphygmomanometer in a busy public area, a five-minute period of rest before pressure determination may not be possible. Just the stress of being in a rush to take the reading, talking, or holding a heavy package may raise the pressure significantly. In addition, cigarette smoking, exercise, and caffeine consumption should be avoided for an hour or more before attempting such a measurement. If the pressure is elevated, the measurement should be repeated one or two more times to determine whether it decreases with time and relaxation. Of course, it may not be practical to make multiple determinations in a busy shopping center.

6 What Is Primary (Essential) Hypertension, and Is It Common?

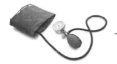

Primary (essential) hypertension is by far the most common type of hypertension. After your doctor excludes the causes of secondary hypertension that can be identified and often corrected (see Question 38), the vast majority of patients are found to have primary hypertension (about 95 percent of all hypertensives). The term *essential* hypertension is a misnomer, because hypertension is not essential for anything. National health surveys suggest that more than 72 million Americans (25 percent of all adults) have systolic blood pressures (BPs) of 140 mm Hg or higher and diastolic BPs of 90 mm Hg or higher. This condition is more common in elderly people and in African Americans. For example, more than 60 percent of African-American women who are over the age of sixty are estimated to have hypertension.

Although the precise cause of primary hypertension remains unknown, this condition is probably the result of multiple factors (see Questions 11, 13, 33). Heredity certainly plays a role in most cases, and more than one genetic abnormality seems to exist. In addition, environmental factors contribute to the development of hypertension. Some individuals are salt sensitive, which means excess salt consumption will elevate their BP. Being overweight or obese, consuming excessive amounts of alcohol, following a sedentary lifestyle, and eating a low-potassium diet may also elevate BP. Although you can't change your genes, gender, age, or racial background, you can certainly avoid environmental factors such as eating too much salt, which may cause or aggravate hypertension. It is noteworthy that healthy lifestyle modifications may not only reduce elevated BP but will also prevent hypertension in a significant segment of the population.

> The cause or causes of primary hypertension are unknown, but both heredity and environmental factors such as salt sensitivity, obesity, consumption of excessive amounts of alcohol, a sedentary lifestyle, and a diet low in potassium can play a role in its development and severity.

To diagnose hypertension, you should conduct your usual activities and take BP readings all through the day while smoking (please quit), working, and relaxing with a martini (just one). If you are diagnosed with hypertension, you will want to monitor your antihypertensive treatment. When doing this, it is better to avoid all possible activities such as drinking coffee, smoking, or exercising that may alter your "baseline" BP for at least one hour prior to taking a reading. Taking one reading before breakfast and coffee and the other prior to drinking any alcohol before dinner is an appropriate schedule for the seven days before your next visit to your doctor.

If the home (and office or schoolroom) readings are being taken to diagnose hypertension, many readings should be taken and recorded, along with the circumstances (e.g., while using the computer, just before dinner.) Take at least twenty sets of readings under various circumstances, some as soon as you wake up, some at work, and some at home before retiring, for example. If most of the readings are at or below 120/80 mm Hg, you are normotensive, even if occasional readings taken under stress, such as while watching your favorite football team get beaten in the Superbowl, are above 140/90 mm Hg.

If the home readings are being taken to monitor your hypertension therapy one week before your next appointment with your doctor, take one set of readings early in the morning and then take another before dinner on each day. Whenever you feel "funny" (e.g., if you feel dizzy when you suddenly get out of bed or if you are bothered by repeated early morning headaches), take your pressure under that condition and note the circumstances in your log book. Be sure to show the readings to your doctor and be sure these readings are considered when deciding upon future management.

7 Why Is High Blood Pressure Bad, and Does Treatment Really Help?

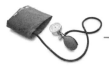

Long ago, insurance companies learned that all applicants for life insurance with high blood pressure above certain levels eventually had more strokes and heart attacks and were more likely to have congestive heart failure, kidney failure, and diseases of the arteries — conditions often leading to disability or premature death — than applicants with normal blood pressures. This fact explains why you cannot get life or disability insurance at standard rates if you have hypertension.

Numerous clinical trials have clearly proved that *patients whose blood pressure is lowered with medication have less risk of stroke, heart attack, and heart failure, as well as a greater probability of a prolonged life when compared with patients who are given placebos* (see Question 74). In fact, these studies have yielded such convincing results that it is now considered unethical to use placebos in trials for more than a short time in almost all patients with hypertension. The ability of newer drugs to control blood pressure and prevent disease complications related to hypertension must now be compared to the activity of older or standard medications (rather than placebo) in trials designed to evaluate their effectiveness.

> *Patients whose blood pressure is lowered with medication have less risk of stroke, heart attack, and heart failure, as well as a greater probability of a prolonged useful life when compared with patients who are given placebos.*

8 What Is the Magnitude of the Hypertension Problem in the United States?

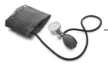

- Hypertension, which can result in stroke, heart attack, heart failure, and kidney failure, is the leading cause of death in the United States, killing almost 1 million people each year. This condition accelerates hardening of the arteries. Other conditions (such as cigarette smoking, abnormal blood lipids, diabetes, obesity, and a sedentary lifestyle) can also contribute to the damaging results of hypertension (see Question 43).

- In the United States, 72 million adults have hypertension—defined as sustained elevations of blood pressure equal to or above 140 mm Hg systolic and/or equal to or above 90 mm Hg diastolic—which means almost one of every three adult Americans has hypertension. Another 45 million have prehypertension (with systolic pressures between 120 and 139 mm Hg and diastolic pressures between 80 and 89 mm Hg), and these people also have an increased risk for developing the disease complications that can result from hypertension.

- Of the 72 million Americans with hypertension, only 50 percent have their BP under control. However, 78 percent of those receiving antihypertensive treatment have their BP controlled, indicating that treatment is highly successful.

- Hypertension is the main cause of invalidism and lost productivity because of brain, heart, and kidney damage. It cripples and disables almost 1 million people each year and is the most common reason people visit a doctor's office.

- The total cost of cardiovascular disease in the United States is over $326 billion annually, with hypertension being a very significant contributor to this expense.

- About one of every four people in the workforce has high blood pressure. One-half of all hypertensives are in the workforce. Hypertension, which can lead to stroke and heart attack, is responsible for the loss of more than 52 million workdays annually.

- More than 75 percent of stroke victims have high blood pressure. Strokes cost Americans more than $45 billion in medical bills and lost earnings each year. The average lifetime medical costs to the patient who suffers a nonfatal stroke are over $140,000.

- Hypertension develops earlier and generally becomes more severe in African Americans than in Caucasians. Stroke and heart disease mortality are 80 percent and 50 percent greater, respectively, and severe hypertensive-related kidney disease occurs five times more often in African Americans than in Caucasians.

- Treating hypertension saves lives and prevents disability!

9 What Are Some Common Misconceptions about Hypertension?

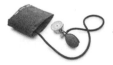

Many people hold a number of misconceptions (or believe in a variety of myths) relating to high blood pressure. Such misinformation deserves correction and clarification, because it can interfere with an individual's proper management of hypertension. The more common and prevalent misconceptions are as follows:

1. Many people with hypertension are convinced that they can tell by the way they feel whether their blood pressure (BP) is elevated. Experience with BP determinations by professionals or by patients who take their BP with twenty-four-hour monitoring devices has shown that patients are usually unable to detect when their BP is high. On the other hand, pain, stress, anxiety, and fear may significantly increase BP in most people regardless of whether they are hypertensive. In addition, some people have "white-coat hypertension" (see Question 14). Under these circumstances, the individual is aware of emotional tension and may correctly guess that BP is elevated, even though no sensation specifically alerts the individual that the pressure is elevated. Feeling very well has nothing to do with BP level and is never an indication that antihypertensive medication should be discontinued. The treatment of hypertension with medication is a lifelong commitment, unless the patient controls their BP by making lifestyle changes and agrees to be monitored.

2. Some people still believe that systolic BP should be roughly 100 plus your age and that BP becomes elevated to maintain adequate flow to the organs of the body. Primary hypertension is the most common form of hypertension (accounting for roughly 95 percent of all cases of elevated blood pressure; see Question 6). In this condition, usually both systolic (the top number) and diastolic (the bottom number) pressures are elevated. Most such cases appear at midlife (thirty-five to fifty

years of age); however, with aging, more individuals develop only systolic hypertension. Despite the fact that the systolic BP often increases with age, the belief that the target reading for systolic BP is 100 plus your age is incorrect.

Elevation of the systolic pressure is increasingly occurring in industrialized countries where most people consume diets that can increase weight and lead to obesity, hardening of the arteries, and hypertension. This higher systolic pressure results from the loss of elasticity of the aorta — the largest artery in the body, which directly receives blood pumped from the heart. As the aorta hardens (becomes arteriosclerotic) with aging, its elasticity (its ability to expand when the heart pumps blood into it) progressively diminishes. As a result, the blood expelled with each contraction (systole) of the heart meets increased resistance because of rigidity in the aorta, and the systolic BP becomes progressively elevated. In native societies, where people are not sedentary and consume little fat, dairy products, or salt, BP and body weight generally do not become elevated with aging. Clearly, then, aging alone does not increase BP. Instead, stiffness of the aorta associated with getting older results largely from poor dietary habits, lack of exercise, and weight gain.

Hypertension never results from the body's effort to improve the circulation of various organs; rather, it reflects an abnormal increase of resistance in large arteries due to atherosclerosis and constriction of small arteries (arterioles). As we all know, hypertension can lead to many negative outcomes (including heart attack, stroke, heart and kidney failure, hardening of the arteries, and, although very rarely, visual impairment). Conversely, lowering BP can prevent or minimize these negative outcomes.

3. Many people believe that hypertension indicates that a person is too tense because of excess stress (see Question 23). In reality, hypertension simply means high BP. Individuals who feel

chronically tense and nervous don't necessarily have higher BPs than people who feel calm and relaxed. Of course, sudden fright, fear, and anxiety can evoke the "fight-or-flight" response, with its ensuing release of epinephrine and activation of the sympathetic nervous system; this response can cause constriction of arteries, which elevates BP. Nevertheless, this natural and temporary response does not result in sustained hypertension.

Significant elevations of BP are encountered in approximately 20 percent of all individuals with normal BPs when their BPs are measured by a doctor. This phenomenon, caused by anxiety, is known as "white-coat hypertension" (see Question 14) because the BP is elevated primarily when in the doctor's presence. Many patients with "white-coat hypertension" will eventually become permanently hypertensive. Consequently, the BPs of individuals with "white-coat hypertension" should be checked more frequently than those of normal subjects in order to identify those most likely to develop sustained hypertension.

4. Some people believe that they can control their BP with lifestyle changes alone. Although reducing excess weight, limiting excess consumption of dietary salt and alcohol, consuming a diet with lots of fruits and vegetables and little saturated fat, and getting adequate exercise may lower elevated BP, antihypertensive medication is usually required to realize optimal BP control. If BP is severely elevated (180/110 mm Hg or greater), antihypertensive drugs are almost always required to achieve optimal control (that is, a BP of 120/80 mm Hg or less). Antihypertensive medication is most effective in persons closely adhering to the lifestyle changes mentioned above and, in these cases, smaller doses of medication are often all that is required. Once the need for antihypertensive medication is recognized, its use is generally ongoing, although with appropriate lifestyle changes — especially considerable weight loss

in obese individuals — it may be possible to reduce or, more rarely, discontinue medication. (See Question 55.)

5. Some people with hypertension believe that they will have to limit their activities. It is prudent for patients with very elevated BP to initially avoid very strenuous exercise, especially weightlifting, as this activity can temporarily elevate BP to dangerous levels. However, regular exercise, such as brisk walking for only thirty minutes daily for most days of the week, is strongly recommended (see Question 46), provided that appropriate testing has ruled out the presence of heart disease. The possible results of hypertension — such as stroke, kidney failure, an aortic aneurysm (a weakened, bulging portion of the aorta), or decreased blood supply to the legs because of atherosclerosis — may, of course, curtail activity. If the individual does not suffer from any of these negative conditions, proper control of BP with antihypertensive drugs and lifestyle changes permit the hypertensive patient to lead a perfectly normal life without curtailing any routine activities.

6. Many people, including some physicians, mistakenly believe that older people (a) comply poorly when taking their medication, (b) do not tolerate their medication very well, and (c) will not benefit much from taking antihypertensive drugs. All of these theories about older people have been proven wrong. In fact, older people take their medication as well, if not better, than younger patients, and treatment is particularly beneficial in the elderly. Smaller doses of medication may be indicated in some older patients, particularly in thin and frail individuals. Nevertheless, with appropriate dosage schedules, older patients tolerate medications and benefit as well as their younger counterparts.

7. Most laypeople and many physicians mistakenly believe that the level of the diastolic BP is far more important than the level of the systolic pressure as a risk determiner for heart attack

and stroke. Years ago, this concept was accepted and widely taught in medical schools. With more experience and scientific study, however, the medical community has found very clearly that the reverse is true—lowering *systolic* pressure is crucial to the prevention of cardiovascular disease and stroke. However, lowering diastolic pressure is also important in preventing the diseases that can result from hypertension.

8. Some patients believe that they can stop taking their antihypertensive medicine when their hypertension is brought under control. Treatment of hypertension merely controls this condition, and it does not cure it. When your doctor tells you that your BP is well controlled, it doesn't mean that you can stop taking the medicine—it means that you must continue to take the medication if you want to keep your BP at a healthy level. Treating hypertension is a lifelong commitment, but it is certainly well worth it.

10 Is There a Personality Type That Is Predisposed to Develop Hypertension?

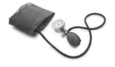

No particular personality type is more likely to develop hypertension than any other. Some psychologists and psychiatrists identify the "hypertensive personality" as rigid, compulsive, and occurring in an individual who cannot openly express hostility. It has been suggested that people with type A personalities—that is, those who are particularly competitive, aggressive, ambitious, and hard-driving—may activate their sympathetic nervous systems, thereby constricting their arteries and causing hypertension and coronary heart disease. However, most hypertensive patients do not have these personality traits. No personality type is immune to the threat of hypertension, and no strong evidence proves that subjects with type A personalities are more likely to develop hypertension than any others.

11 Is Primary (Essential) Hypertension Inherited?

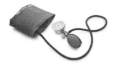

Primary hypertension may be inherited and frequently runs in families — but so do other unhealthy characteristics and lifestyles (such as obesity, heavy alcohol consumption, a sedentary lifestyle, and poor dietary habits). Blood pressure usually increases with increasing weight, and almost 50 percent of obese people have high blood pressure. If one parent has primary hypertension, his or her child has a 50 percent chance of developing hypertension; this risk increases to almost 100 percent if both parents are hypertensive. Much research is now devoted to identifying genes that might cause high blood pressure. Most likely, multiple genes will be implicated because it is unlikely that nearly all patients with hypertension share the same genetic abnormalities. For example, up to 60 percent of hypertensive individuals are salt sensitive — but the other 40 percent are not. Furthermore, the incidence of hypertension among African Americans may be at least twice that observed among whites. Clearly, the cause of primary hypertension is complex and influenced by multiple factors (see Question 6).

> *Primary hypertension may be inherited and frequently runs in families—but so do other unhealthy characteristics and lifestyles.*

12 What Is "Mild Hypertension"?

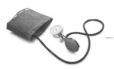

The term "mild hypertension" has increasingly been discarded, because it is misleading. While it is true that the higher the blood pressure (BP), the greater the risk of negative health consequences, even patients with "mild hypertension" (with systolic blood pressures in the vicinity of 140 mm Hg and diastolic pressures near 90 mm Hg) are at increased risk of having

> *The term "mild hypertension" has increasingly been discarded, because it is misleading.*

a stroke, heart attack, heart failure, or kidney failure, although those events may take longer to develop or occur. The *Seventh Report of the Joint National Committee on Prevention, Detection, Evaluation, and Treatment of High Blood Pressure (JNC7)* recommends using "stages" of hypertension, rather than the old terminology of "mild," "moderate," and "severe" (see Table 1).

Table 1. Classification of Blood Pressure for Adults Age Eighteen and Older*

Category	Systolic (mmHg)		Diastolic (mmHg)
Optimal**	<120	and	<80
Prehypertension	>120	or	>80, <90
Hypertension***			
Stage 1	140–159	or	90–99
Stage 2	>160		>100

> means greater than   < means less than

* Not taking antihypertensive drugs and not acutely ill. Isolated systolic hypertension is defined as systolic BP of 140 mm Hg or greater and diastolic BP of less than 90 mm Hg. In addition to classifying stages of hypertension on the basis of average BP levels, clinicians should indicate the presence or absence of target organ disease and additional risk factors. This information is important for risk classification and treatment.

** Optimal BP with respect to cardiovascular risk is less than 120/80 mm Hg, but unusually low readings should be evaluated for clinical significance.

*** Diagnosis based on an average of two or more readings taken at each of two or more visits following an initial screening.

13 What Mechanisms Cause Hypertension?

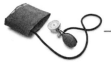

Blood pressure (BP) is dependent on the heart rate, the amount of blood pumped with each beat, and the degree of constriction in the arterioles. Other factors such as the amount of blood in the circulation and even the thickness of the blood (which largely depends on the number of red blood cells in the circulation) can also influence the BP.

It is important to understand that BP may vary considerably during the day and can be influenced by many conditions. Conditions that increase the pumping force of the heart — such as exercise, some drugs and hormones, or increased blood volume — can increase the amount of blood pumped with each heartbeat and hence elevate BP, particularly the systolic pressure (which occurs during contraction of the heart). Hardening of the large arteries (arteriosclerosis) may also increase systolic pressure.

On the other hand, conditions that activate the sympathetic nervous system — such as stimulation of the nervous system, neurohormones, certain drugs, severe anxiety, or a very cold temperature — and stimulate vascular smooth muscles, promote constriction of arterioles. This constriction also elevates BP, primarily the diastolic

> *Conditions that increase the pumping force of the heart can increase the amount of blood pumped with each heartbeat and hence elevate BP, particularly the systolic pressure. Conditions that activate the sympathetic nervous system and stimulate vascular smooth muscles can cause constriction of arterioles and also elevate BP, primarily the diastolic pressure.*

pressure (the pressure when the heart is not contracting, which mainly depends on the degree of constriction of the arterioles). Occasionally, with sudden fear and anxiety (the "fight-or-flight" reaction), increased pumping force of the heart and constriction of arterioles may occur together and boost BP. Even normal individuals periodically have hypertensive BP elevations during the day (see Question 36). These transitory elevations pose no serious risk unless the BP becomes extremely high.

Primary hypertension, which accounts for the hypertension found in about 95 percent of all hypertensive patients, exists when elevations in BP are sustained without any identifiable cause. Genetics can certainly play a role in this condition's development, as the condition is much more common in the offspring of parents who have hypertension; multiple hypertension-related genetic abnormalities appear to exist. Perhaps 60 percent of people with primary hypertension are salt sensitive; that is, excessive salt consumption causes hypertension in these individuals (see Question 34). Exactly why salt produces hypertension remains unclear. Salt retention by the kidneys of people with salt sensitivity may be accompanied by increased body fluid and blood volume that initially might play a role in elevating BP; however, *the main abnormality responsible for the elevated BP observed in primary hypertension appears to be increased constriction of the arterioles, the cause of which remains unknown.*

The causes of secondary hypertension, which accounts for only 5 percent of all hypertensive patients, are known and are discussed in detail in Question 38. Some of these causes are damaged kidneys or functional impairment, hormonal tumors, and other endocrine abnormalities. In particular, a variety of drugs and hormones, any conditions that stimulate the nervous system, preeclampsia or eclampsia during pregnancy, coarctation (constriction) of the aorta, and sleep apnea can cause or exacerbate hypertension. In these conditions, the hypertension may result from increased constriction of the arterioles, increased pumping force of the heart, or both. The hypertension in coarctation (a narrowing of the aorta, the large artery carrying blood from the heart to the upper and lower body) occurs only in the upper part of the body and is mainly due to the blockage of blood flow caused by coarctation; impaired blood flow to the kidneys resulting from the coarctation may, however, also produce a chemical substance that constricts arterioles.

Hypertension is, therefore, a manifestation of an increased resistance to blood flow because of constriction of arterioles, or occasionally an increased output of blood by the heart, or a combination of these changes. As indicated above, a large number of conditions and diseases may be responsible for these changes that produce hypertension.

14 What Is "White-coat" or "Masked" Hypertension? Do I Have Either, and Are They Dangerous?

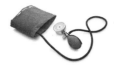

"White-coat hypertension" is hypertension that occurs when blood pressure (BP) is measured by a doctor. With this condition, BP remains normal when measured by the patient or by others at home, in the workplace, or elsewhere (see Question 19) — consistently measuring more than 10 mm Hg lower than the office readings. According to the late Dr. Thomas Pickering, a specialist in hypertension who had extensively studied this type of hypertension, 20 percent of patients who had elevated BP when measured by the doctor in his or her office

> "White-coat hypertension" is hypertension that occurs when blood pressure is taken by the doctor; blood pressure remains normal when measured by the patient or by others at home, in the workplace, or elsewhere.

subsequently had relatively normal BPs (below 135/85 mm Hg) when they were electronically monitored for twenty-four hours.

Although white-coat hypertension may affect anyone, it is slightly more common in women than in men. It occurs in approximately 40 percent of individuals older than sixty-five who have hypertension when BP is determined by the doctor. No evidence suggests that people with white-coat hypertension have a certain personality type or are more neurotic than anyone else; furthermore, their BP reacts to a variety of stresses in the same way as does the BP of individuals without white-coat hypertension. It appears that the doctor (the "white-coat" figure) engenders a significant sense of fear and anxiety in certain patients, sometimes even accompanied by an increase in heart rate, which results in an abnormal increase in BP. This reaction probably reflects some apprehension that the doctor may report bad news; that is, that the patient's BP is elevated. This threat may persist for years when BP is measured by the doctor, despite a prolonged and friendly relationship with the physician.

White-coat hypertension requires that the BP be in the hypertensive range (greater than 140/90 mm Hg) when recorded by the doctor on several office visits but consistently normal when recorded out of the office. For accurate BP determinations, it is important that the patient remains seated and relaxed in a quiet environment for at least five minutes; that the individual avoids exercise, smoking, and drinks containing caffeine for one hour before the recording; and that the patient avoids stress of any type just prior to the measurement. BP may be taken frequently throughout the day by the patient or other individuals, or it may be monitored every fifteen minutes for twenty-four hours and recorded by an automatic electronic device. (Note: BP–reading machines in pharmacies and shopping areas may not always be accurate for these readings. See Question 5.)

BP over the entire twenty-four hours, including sleep, can be measured with ambulatory BP monitoring (ABPM). Such monitoring, although it adds greatly to and shortens considerably the assessment of BP, is not frequently performed in the United States, because third-party payers (such as Medicare and private insurance companies) will usually not pay for the procedure.

Patients who are truly hypertensive will have elevated BP no matter who takes the measurement and no matter where it is taken. Of course, hypertensive patients may also be apprehensive when the doctor measures their BP and, therefore, also may have somewhat higher BP in that circumstance than when pressure is measured by someone outside the doctor's office.

It remains unclear whether individuals with white-coat hypertension are more likely to develop sustained hypertension and the negative health outcomes associated with it than are people whose BP remains less than 140/90 mm Hg, both inside and outside the doctor's office. Usually antihypertensive medication is not recommended for people with white-coat hypertension if the condition has not damaged the heart, brain, or blood vessels elsewhere, although a healthy lifestyle is clearly appropriate.

People with white-coat hypertension should have their BP measured every few months to verify that persistent hypertension has not developed, as some evidence suggests that these patients have a greater chance of developing hypertension than normal subjects. Furthermore, it is recommended that patients with white-coat hypertension, if indicated, lose excess weight, limit salt and alcohol consumption, stop smoking, and undertake adequate aerobic exercise. Adhering to the DASH eating plan (see page 95) will help reduce weight and limit salt consumption. Checking the BP frequently — at least several times each year — and making any necessary lifestyle changes will ensure the proper management of patients with this type of hypertension, since some of these patients may develop stroke and heart disease.

The late Dr. Thomas Pickering was the first to identify "masked" or "reverse" hypertension. This condition is exactly the opposite of white-coat hypertension; that is, normal BP readings are recorded in the doctor's office but high readings occur when the BP is measured elsewhere. This pattern has been noted in 10 to 20 percent of adults and obviously requires multiple out-of-office readings to identify "masked hypertension." If present, it should be treated as if the patient has sustained hypertension, since these patients are at risk for developing stroke, heart, and kidney disease.

15 What Are the Purposes of the Pretreatment Examination?

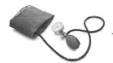

There are four main reasons why patients with hypertension should be evaluated before starting treatment:

1. to identify patients who have a curable cause for their high blood pressure
2. to assess the status of the affected parts of the body: the heart, brain, eyes, kidneys, and blood vessels
3. to identify other cardiovascular risk factors — for example, diabetes, smoking, high serum cholesterol, age, upper-body

obesity, a sedentary lifestyle, a family history of premature stroke or heart attack—that could affect the need for and the choice of treatment

4. to ensure that the elevated blood pressure is sustained over a period of time; that is, to rule out "white-coat hypertension" caused by anxiety in the presence of the doctor (see Question 14)

The tests that a doctor may order to get this information are discussed in Question 16.

16 What Tests Will My Doctor Order Before I Start Taking Medication for My High Blood Pressure? Are an Echocardiogram and Stress Test Necessary?

Not everyone who has high blood pressure needs medication. The purpose of the examination is to aid the physician in deciding whether you need only medication, only lifestyle changes, or a combination of the two. For patients who have Stage 1 hypertension (see Table 1 on page 20; also see Question 12) but show no evidence of target organ disease (that is, no apparent heart, brain, kidney, or visual damage) and have no other risk factors (such as male sex, cigarette smoking, blood lipid abnormalities, diabetes, obesity, or a sedentary lifestyle), medication might be appropriately withheld until the full benefits of lifestyle modifications can be achieved.

The purpose of the examination is to aid the physician in deciding whether you need only medication, only lifestyle changes, or a combination of the two.

Usually an electrocardiogram is recommended to evaluate the heart. Blood tests help rule out diabetes mellitus; they evaluate your cholesterol levels, including levels of LDL (low-density lipoprotein, or "bad" cholesterol) and HDL (high-density lipoprotein, or "good" cholesterol), as well as your triglyceride level (another type of lipid) — that is, fats that may damage blood vessels and cause heart disease. A urinalysis is essential to detect kidney disease; albumin in the urine is a particularly important sign of kidney disease.

Some doctors may not agree, but it seems prudent to also determine concentrations of homocysteine and C-reactive protein (CRP) in the blood of patients who have any evidence of damage to the brain, heart, kidney, or blood vessels. Homocysteine (a substance in the body used to make proteins) may contribute to the hardening of the arteries (atherosclerosis) and increase the risk of stroke and heart disease. Although the role homocysteine plays in causing blood vessel damage is unclear, it seems reasonable to reduce an elevated homocysteine by increasing consumption of folic acid and vitamins B-6 and B-12. Elevated CRP may be an indication of inflammation, atherosclerosis, heart failure, and hypertension. It may also possibly contribute to the formation of atherosclerosis and hypertension. Some drugs used to treat diabetes, lower bad cholesterol in the blood, or prevent the formation of angiotensin may lower concentrations of CRP in the blood. However, whether lowering CRP in the blood has a beneficial effect on health is unclear.

Creatinine determinations can be helpful in determining the degree of impaired kidney function. Finally, determination of uric acid is indicated in the presence of impaired kidney function since some evidence suggests that uric acid may cause damage to small blood vessels and possibly play a role in the development of hypertension.

Multiple readings of blood pressure both in the office and sometimes in the home are necessary to establish a baseline and to exclude the possibility of "white-coat hypertension" (see Question 14) before any treatment is prescribed. A physical examination is important to identify target organ disease or curable secondary causes of high blood pressure. In addition, a urinalysis is helpful to evaluate the kidney as a target organ or possible kidney disease as a cause of the hypertension. All of this information aids your physician in determining appropriate treatment.

An echocardiogram is usually not necessary. The electrocardiogram (ECG), which reveals the electrical activity of the heart, is much simpler to perform, and it usually provides the information needed for evaluating the heart prior to treatment. In some cases, and especially when heart failure is suspected, an echocardiogram, which visualizes the size, configuration, and pumping force of the heart, provides more detailed information than the electrocardiogram. The echocardiogram is much more sensitive in detecting early evidence of enlargement and thickening of the walls of the heart, but it is a much more expensive test. Enlargement of the heart sometimes accompanies hypertension and may require more aggressive treatment.

A chest X ray also may be ordered, especially if the patient has not received one for many years, just to confirm that no abnormalities of the lungs or heart are present. If the patient has had hypertension for a long time, the X ray may reveal enlargement of the heart, especially the left ventricle, which, as the main pumping chamber of the heart, has to pump against the elevated pressure.

A stress test, in which the electrocardiogram is recorded during exercise, is not routinely ordered. However, if there is any sensation or feeling of chest pressure or pain that might be due to coronary artery disease, then a stress test is usually indicated. It is prudent for postmenopausal women and men over the age of forty-five to take a stress test to detect any impaired circulation in the heart, especially for those people planning to begin an exercise program.

17 Is a "Renin Profile" Necessary to Treat My Hypertension?

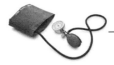

A renin profile is not necessary to begin hypertension treatment. The renin profile measures an enzyme called renin in the blood.

Physicians had hoped that the serum concentration of renin (which generates a hypertensive substance called angiotensin) would predict which medications would be the most appropriate and effective for a given patient since they found that, in general, patients with low-renin hypertension respond well to diuretics, whereas those with high-renin hypertension respond well to angiotensin-converting enzyme (ACE) inhibitors, angiotensin receptor blockers (ARBs), or direct renin inhibitors. Unfortunately, the renin profile has not proved to be a valuable therapeutic guide; it is unnecessary and can even be misleading. Insurance companies will not pay for it either. In special circumstances, determination of the blood's renin level may help identify patients in whom hypertension results from excess production of renin by the kidney; very low levels of renin sometimes indicates the presence of an adrenal tumor.

18 Do I Need to See a Specialist to Have My Hypertension Treated?

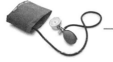

The vast majority of hypertensive patients are treated by primary-care physicians who are knowledgeable about the variety of drugs available to treat the condition. The reasons for a referral to a specialist might include the following:

- difficulty keeping your blood pressure controlled to less than 140/90 mm Hg most of the time without side effects from medication
- complications of hypertension (i.e., negative health effects stemming from hypertension)
- multiple risk factors in addition to hypertension

If a secondary cause of hypertension is suspected, consultation with a hypertension specialist may help establish the diagnosis and lead to the appropriate management tactics for the rarer causes of elevated blood pressure.

19 Are Measurements of Blood Pressure at Home Important in Managing Hypertension, and Should I Have My Blood Pressure Monitored for Twenty-four Hours?

Home blood pressure (BP) measurements can be extremely valuable in the management of hypertension (see Question 14). A twenty-four-hour monitoring of your BP by an electronic device is rarely necessary for diagnosis and treatment.

Home BP measurements offer three major advantages:

1. They can establish whether elevated BP in the doctor's office involves "white-coat hypertension" due to emotional tension from anxiety and fear surrounding the visit to the doctor (see Question 14).

2. They enable your physician to evaluate the effectiveness of antihypertensive medications and to make appropriate adjustments in dosage.

3. They may identify patients with "masked" or "reverse" hypertension who need to initiate a healthy lifestyle (if indicated) and/or start antihypertensive medication.

> *Although home blood pressure measurements can be extremely valuable in the management of hypertension, twenty-four-hour monitoring of blood pressure by an electronic device is rarely necessary for diagnosis and treatment.*

In addition, the discipline required to keep records of home-measured BPs and periodically report these results can lead to a stronger patient–doctor relationship and help ensure that patients continue taking their medication. Taking your BP a few times each week should be adequate. Finally, the need for office visits may be very significantly reduced, providing considerable savings to the patient in terms of medical expenses and the time and inconvenience of office visits.

Almost all patients can measure their BP at home. We suggest that patients use an electronic sphygmomanometer that simply requires the cuff be placed around the arm in the usual way (see

Question 3); with the press of a button, the cuff automatically inflates and deflates, giving the systolic and diastolic BP readings as well as the heart rate. Most electronic sphygmomanometers are highly accurate; nevertheless, their accuracy should be periodically validated by comparing their BP determinations with those obtained with the doctor's office sphygmomanometer. An extra-large cuff should be used for obese patients or patients with large, muscular arms.

When measuring BP at home, the patient should remember to remain seated, at rest, and relaxed in a quiet environment for at least a few minutes before the measurement. Smoking, caffeine, and exercise should be avoided for one hour before taking the reading, and any stress should be avoided just prior to the measurement. Even talking can increase systolic and diastolic pressure, so BP measurements should be made while the patient is not speaking. Another reason for using an electronic sphygmomanometer is that no physical activity is required to inflate the cuff, as even this small activity might increase BP. Because BP readings are usually higher in the early morning than in the afternoon or evening, it is helpful to record BPs periodically at different times of the day when starting a new treatment; the results may indicate the need for administering some medications more than once daily.

Home-based measurements of BP have increased in popularity in recent years and are strongly recommended. They are a reliable guide for physicians treating hypertensive patients, and they correlate well with target organ damage such as enlargement of the left ventricle of the heart (the main pumping chamber) and the occurrence of kidney damage. Note, however, that BP measurements taken throughout a twenty-four-hour period more accurately reveal target organ damage involving the heart, kidney, eyes, and carotid arteries (the arteries that supply blood to the brain).

As previously mentioned, twenty-four-hour ambulatory BP monitoring can help identify patients with suspected "white-coat hypertension" (see Question 14) and in assessing the effectiveness of antihypertensive treatment. In addition, it can prove especially valuable in linking symptoms of very low BP to antihypertensive treatment and in correlating symptoms of an excessive excitation of the sympathetic nervous system with excessive release of hormones (epinephrine and norepinephrine) into the circulation with episodic hypertension accompanied by a rapid heart rate, profuse sweating, and headache (see Question 35). Likewise, twenty-four-hour monitoring may supply important information about individuals thought to be suffering from sleep apnea. This type of monitoring is not usually needed in the management of hypertension.

20 Which Blood Pressure Is More Important—Systolic or Diastolic?

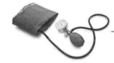

It now appears that elevated systolic pressure puts one at a greater risk for developing negative health effects than elevated diastolic pressure (see Question 2). For many years, diastolic blood pressure was considered more important, probably because the blood vessels are subjected to this type of pressure most of the time (between heartbeats). Recently, however, observational studies have concluded that the systolic blood pressure is actually a much better predictor of strokes, heart attacks, heart failure, kidney disease, and overall mortality.

> *Elevated systolic pressure puts one at a greater risk for developing negative health effects than elevated diastolic pressure.*

Elevation of only the systolic pressure (isolated systolic hypertension) occurs quite frequently in older individuals and usually results from a "hardening" (arteriosclerosis) of the large arteries. This physical change may be accompanied by significant arteriosclerosis in the arteries of the heart and brain, which increases the likelihood of stroke and heart attack. Elevated diastolic pressure is less accurate than systolic pressure as a predictor of negative health outcomes stemming from hypertension, especially in patients over age fifty.

21 Is High Blood Pressure Mostly in the Arteries, or Can It Also Occur in Veins?

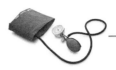

The high blood pressure that is discussed in this book is "arterial hypertension"; that is, high blood pressure in the arteries going to all parts of the body except the lungs. Pressure in the veins, which is normally much lower than pressure in the arteries, is not affected in this type of hypertension, although it may sometimes be high due to heart failure or obstruction of the veins (not related to arterial hypertension). This fact undoubtedly explains why the damage from high blood pressure occurs in the arteries and not in the veins.

> *"Arterial hypertension" involves high blood pressure in the arteries.*

To refresh your memory, arteries carry blood from the heart to the organs and tissues, which are in return fed by tiny, microscopic vessels called capillaries. The arterioles (the smallest arteries) are microscopic, muscular extensions of the arteries found before the arterial system breaks up into capillaries (see Question 1). Most authorities believe that high blood pressure occurs because of greater-than-normal constriction of the arterioles, which produces resistance to the flow of blood in the arteries. The veins are thin-walled vessels that return blood from the tissues to the heart and lungs; they are not affected by hypertension.

22 Is It Normal for Blood Pressure to Increase with Age?

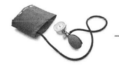

In the United States and other industrialized societies such as Western Europe, blood pressure (BP) *does* increase with age, but this does not necessarily make it "normal." In less industrialized (more native) societies, such as Indian tribes in the Amazon jungles of Brazil and inhabitants of remote regions of the South Pacific, BP stays low (by Western standards) throughout life. The Western lifestyle — which is characterized by unhealthy diet, excess weight, and limited physical activity — may be responsible for the tendency of BP to increase with age. "Low BP" populations are characterized by diets low in saturated fat and salt, vigorous exercise, a lean body weight throughout life, and a lack of exposure to industrialization, which to some implies a more tranquil lifestyle.

The BP of infants at the time of birth is less than 100/60 mm Hg in both civilized and native societies. In the native societies, BP does rise but is rarely above 100/60 mm Hg, without further elevation throughout life. In the United States, it is considered "normal" for BP to rise during the first twenty years of life. This measurement is not considered "high" until it exceeds 136/87 mm Hg for seventeen-year-old boys of average height; for girls, BP is slightly less. Because of progressive "hardening" (arteriosclerosis) of the large arteries, systolic BP tends to increase with age throughout life for both men and women in the United States. This "average" increase should not be considered normal — the progressive elevation of BP accounts for the high morbidity and mortality rate from cardiovascular disease in elderly Americans. The old adage that systolic BP should be 100 plus your age is both unhealthy and untrue. The average diastolic BP in the United States tends to increase until a person is between fifty and fifty-five years of age; after that it then begins to decline. It is noteworthy that adolescents from acculturated societies who die from accidental trauma may have early evidence of hardening of the arteries even without elevated BP or cholesterol. An unhealthy lifestyle may be responsible.

> *The old adage that systolic blood pressure should be 100 plus your age is both unhealthy and untrue.*

23 Can Stress Cause Hypertension, and How Can You Reduce Stress?

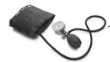

Although some people think that hypertension means that they are "hyper-tense," in reality hypertension simply means "high blood pressure (BP)." Nevertheless, emotional tension or stress can result from unpleasant physical or mental stimuli and is usually associated with a transitory increase in heart and respiratory rates and BP (see Question 9). This is a normal response — one that we all experience — and the BP and heart and breathing rates return to their original rates after removal of stress. The notion that stress is a *major* cause of *permanent* hypertension is incorrect.

> The notion that stress is a major cause of permanent hypertension is incorrect.

All humans experience stressful events in their lives, and the resulting release of hormones by the adrenal glands can be valuable in increasing alertness, fueling the competitive drive, and enhancing athletic and job performance. The response to various types of stress differs from person to person. For example, the anxiety and emotional stress of having one's BP taken by a doctor causes 20 percent of patients to experience "white-coat hypertension" (see Question 14). Although stress can trigger a "fight-or-flight" reaction occasioned by anticipation of physical conflict, the response can vary significantly in different individuals. While the response to stress is usually greater in men than in women, the stress response to a crying baby has been reported to be greater in women than it is in men.

One investigator reported some fascinating observations of BP change, which he recorded frequently with an electronic device during a twenty-four-hour period. Even talking on the telephone was found to raise the systolic BP 5 mm Hg; in contrast, relaxing or watching television caused the pressure to drop. In this study, the highest BP measurements were recorded at work or during commuting. In the evening after work, unmarried women usually experienced a decrease in pressure; the BP in married women with children did not decrease during this time. Men's BP usually declined in the evening regardless of whether they had children. It was suggested that women with young children have two causes of stress: (1) their jobs during the day and (2) their family responsibilities during the evening. Nevertheless, no evidence indicates that women who have full-time jobs during the day and a family to care for in the evening are more likely to develop hypertension.

Although it might seem reasonable to believe that repeated, pronounced elevations of BP can damage blood vessels and increase the occurrence of stroke and heart attack, there is no strong evidence confirming this occurrence in people with normal BP. Furthermore, no evidence indicates that people with type A personalities (highly competitive, ambitious, aggressive, impatient, perfectionistic) are more prone to hypertension than other people (see Question 10). Some studies have found that men with stressful jobs over which they have no control are more prone to eventually develop hypertension and experience heart attacks, especially if they are blue-collar workers with limited education. Particularly noteworthy is the finding that air traffic controllers, who are exposed to considerable psychological stress, develop hypertension at a rate five to six times greater than do pilots who share similar physical characteristics. In addition, men who are constantly striving to improve their lifestyle status and live beyond their financial means are more likely to develop hypertension than men who remain content with their status quo. But it is not clear whether it is the stress or the accompanying unhealthy lifestyle these people adopt, which includes increased alcohol, food, and salt consumption, a lack of exercise, and a resulting weight gain, that contribute to their elevated BP. In contrast, people living in protected and secluded societies (for example, nuns) have been found to maintain relatively low BP readings throughout life. But here, too, it may be that their lifestyles and diets may aid in protecting them from elevated BP. In individuals with hypertension, stress may further aggravate hypertension and increase the risk of arterial damage, stroke, and heart attack.

Clearly, some people define and handle stress much better than others. The response to stress depends on the amount and type of stress and on its duration. Under certain circumstances, prolonged psychological stress may contribute to the development of sustained hypertension in some individuals.

As mentioned earlier, a sudden and very stressful event may cause severe anxiety accompanied by a pronounced increase in BP and heart rate accompanied by excess perspiration. This response ends when the stress is removed. Occasionally, however, a sudden rise in BP and heart rate may cause an irregular heartbeat, pain or a pressure sensation in the chest (angina), and even a heart attack in people with impaired circulation in the heart.

In contrast, chronic stress may result in fatigue, irritability, headaches, an inability to concentrate, insomnia, depression, discouragement, frequent complaints, and unhappiness. Work performance may be disrupted, and family life can suffer disastrous consequences. Chronic stress may make an individual feel trapped with no way out, no escape hatch. Furthermore, it may suppress the immune system and make an individual more susceptible to infections and malignant tumors. Nevertheless, chronic stress does not cause persistent hypertension.

The management of stress, which recurs on a daily basis, can be difficult. The following basic steps may prove very helpful in this regard:

- **Getting adequate sleep — at least seven hours each night — is important.** Over-the-counter sleep medication (usually a pain reliever plus an antihistamine, such as Tylenol PM) may be very helpful. Prescription drugs are rarely indicated to induce sleep; they can be habit forming and should only be used as directed by a doctor.

- **Eating a healthy and moderate-sized meal at least two hours before retiring and consuming no more than one or two alcoholic drinks with the evening meal is recommended.** Consuming a large meal and drinking excessive alcohol may interfere with sleep.

- **Getting adequate aerobic exercise (thirty minutes per day, most days per week) on a regular basis is critical.** Exercise is not only good for your physical condition, but it can also have a remarkably beneficial effect on emotional tension. Physical conditioning and maintaining appropriate weight may improve your appearance, make you feel good about yourself, and relieve some of the stress that may result from inactivity and being overweight.

• **Finding other avenues of stress relief.** Of some interest are reports that some individuals who develop a strong attachment and warm affection for pets (for example, dogs and cats) find these animals can relieve stress and lower BP.

> *Avoiding conflict, maintaining a positive attitude, scheduling work to avoid being rushed at the last minute, avoiding inessential duties, getting adequate vacation time, and pursuing muscle relaxation techniques, meditation, and biofeedback may prove beneficial in stress management.*

Avoiding conflict, getting adequate vacation time, maintaining a positive attitude, scheduling work to avoid being rushed at the last minute, avoiding inessential duties, and pursuing muscle relaxation techniques, meditation, and biofeedback may prove beneficial in stress management and could be an adjunct to therapy. Unfortunately, these tactics alone are usually ineffective in controlling chronic hypertension. If stress continues and becomes intolerable, psychiatric consultation and drugs that reduce tension without significantly impairing performance may be appropriate.

24 Does Alcohol Increase Blood Pressure? How Much Can I Drink If I Have Hypertension?

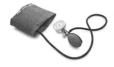

Seven to 10 percent of all cases of hypertension in the United States are caused by excess alcohol consumption. This percentage is considerably higher in communities and countries in which many individuals regularly drink alcohol in excessive amounts.

Men who have hypertension and who also consume alcohol

should limit their intake to no more than two ounces of 80- to 100-proof spirits, two cans of beer, or two glasses of wine each day (equivalent to 1 ounce of ethanol). Women or small men should limit their intake to half this amount. Restricting alcohol consumption is especially important for hypertensive women, because they have less of the enzyme alcohol dehydrogenase (an enzyme important for metabolizing alcohol) in their stomach than men. The moderate amount of alcohol consumption recommended here rarely

> Men who have hypertension and who also consume alcohol should limit their intake to no more than two ounces of 80- to 100-proof spirits, two cans of beer, or two glasses of wine each day. Women or small men should limit their intake to half this amount.

causes an elevation of blood pressure (BP) and even appears to decrease the occurrence of heart attacks when compared to teetotalers. If you have hypertension and find that even this moderate consumption of alcohol increases your BP, then you should not drink alcohol.

Note that alcohol consumption provides a significant number of calories (one bottle of beer contains 100 to 150 calories, and one glass of wine contains about 125 calories) without any nutritional benefit. This point is worth remembering if you are hypertensive and trying to lose weight. Modest alcohol intake may elevate the level of "good" cholesterol (high-density lipoprotein [HDL]), which protects arteries from accumulating cholesterol deposits. Nevertheless, alcohol consumption should certainly be limited in hypertensive individuals.

There is evidence that consumption of red wine may protect individuals from heart attacks. Although the explanation for this effect remains unclear, a chemical in the wine that decreases the tendency of blood to clot may play a role. Before endorsing the consumption of red or white wine, one should take heed of the fact that excess consumption of wine in France accounts for the highest incidence of cirrhosis (liver disease) in the world. Once again, moderation in wine consumption is the key.

The reason why excess alcohol elevates BP is uncertain. The lower BP associated with a reduction of excess alcohol consumption can be impressive — systolic and diastolic pressure may decrease as much as 13 mm Hg and 7 mm Hg, respectively. If a heavy drinker wishes to curtail his or her alcohol consumption, this reduction should occur gradually. Abrupt cessation of alcohol intake can stimulate the sympathetic nervous system by liberating hormones (epinephrine and norepinephrine), which can then constrict arteries and sometimes cause severe hypertension. Heavy drinkers should consult a physician and develop a program for cessation of drinking so as to minimize or prevent symptoms of alcohol withdrawal such as anxiety, shakiness, insomnia, upset stomach, and increased pulse, temperature, and respiration. Some heavy drinkers may also experience confusion and hallucinations as they go through withdrawal.

Finally, it should be noted that alcohol consumption in addition to its effect on coordination, reflex reaction time, and judgment, may enhance the effect of some antihypertensive medications, leading to a decrease in BP that may cause one to feel faint and unsteady. This interaction could be particularly hazardous while driving a car.

25 Does High Blood Pressure Occur in Children, and Should Children and Adolescents with Primary Hypertension Be Treated?

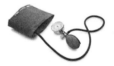

High blood pressure (BP) does indeed occur in children — and more frequently than we thought, at least until pediatricians started measuring BP in children on routine office visits. Remember that "normal" BP for children is lower than it is in adults. For instance, at age one year, the upper limit of "normal" is 104/58 mm Hg for a girl of average height and 102/57 mm Hg for a boy of average height. By age seventeen, these upper limits of normal have increased to 129/84 mm Hg for a girl and 136/87 mm Hg for a boy. Pediatricians believe that BP in children should be related to their height. Most pediatric hypertension is related to increased weight, and pediatricians prefer to manage hypertension in children and adolescents with lifestyle modifications, if possible. Such a strategy includes weight reduction when the patient is obese, reduction of sodium in the diet to no more than 2,400 mg per day, and adequate aerobic exercise. Hypertensive children and adolescents should avoid excess dietary fat and the "fast food" that many in this age group so frequently consume. Hypertension should not restrict children's participation in sports, unless the BP is very high. After the BP has been successfully lowered, exercise can prove very beneficial.

> *Pediatricians prefer to manage hypertension in children and adolescents with lifestyle modifications, if possible. If these measures fail, drugs are recommended with an appropriate modification of the dosage depending upon the patient's body weight.*

If these measures fail to modify the hypertension, drugs are recommended with an appropriate modification of the dosage depending upon the patient's body weight. ACE inhibitors, angiotensin receptor blockers, and direct renin inhibitors should not be prescribed for pregnant or sexually active girls (see Question 66).

Finally, it is important to recognize that hypertension in children and adolescents, particularly if severe, is often due to secondary causes (see Question 38).

26 Does Hypertension Affect White and African-American Individuals Differently?

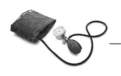

African Americans of any age are more likely to have hypertension than their white counterparts. Not only does hypertension occur more frequently in the African-American population, but it is often more severe. In addition, African-American individuals are more likely to have complications earlier in the course of the disease. The mortality rate for stroke is 80 percent higher and the mortality rate for heart disease is 50 percent higher in African Americans than in whites. Kidney complications marked by kidney failure are five times more frequently observed in African Americans than in whites.

The explanation for the greater prevalence and severity of hypertension in African Americans than in white individuals remains unclear. However, approximately 60 percent of hypertensive people are salt sensitive (see Question 34); that is, their blood pressure becomes significantly elevated when they consume excess amounts of table salt (sodium chloride). Salt sensitivity may result from a genetic kidney abnormality that causes the retention of excess amounts of sodium, an abnormality that is especially common in African Americans. Excess salt consumption by individuals who are salt sensitive will, of course, aggravate hypertension and its severity.

> *African Americans of any age are more likely to have hypertension than their white counterparts. Not only does hypertension occur more frequently in the African-American population, but it is often more severe.*

27 What Is Malignant Hypertension?

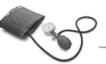

"Malignant hypertension"—the most severe form of hypertension—is rapidly progressive and leads quickly to target organ damage. Unless properly treated, it is fatal within five years for about 90 percent of its victims. Death usually comes from congestive heart failure, kidney failure, or brain hemorrhage.

Patients with malignant hypertension characteristically demonstrate tiny hemorrhages and exudates (white spots) in the retina at the back of the eyes. The optic nerve seen in the back of each eye may be swollen (papilledema). Fortunately, aggressive treatment can reverse

> *"Malignant hypertension"—the most severe form of hypertension—is rapidly progressive and leads quickly to target organ damage. Unless properly treated, it is fatal within five years for about 90 percent of its victims.*

malignant hypertension and prevent it from leading to negative health results. In fact, this type of hypertension is now quite rare, whereas thirty or forty years ago (before the advent of effective drugs) it was much more common. Malignant hypertension is not attributable to cancer or a malignancy, although, if untreated, it will cause a rapidly fatal outcome.

28 Why Is Primary (Essential) Hypertension Called "The Silent Killer"? Is It a Disease?

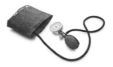

In one sense, it is unfortunate that the most common type of high blood pressure (BP) — primary hypertension — very rarely causes symptoms or signs that warn individuals about their elevated BP. As a consequence, disease complications from hypertension, including hardening of the arteries, stroke, heart attack, heart and kidney failure, impaired vision, and death may occur before the BP elevation is recognized — hence the name "the silent killer." Many people believe that a red or flushed appearance of the face is always a sign of hypertension and that a headache is a common symptom of an elevated BP; these notions are actually misconceptions (see Question 9). Mild headaches may occasionally affect some hypertensives, but only rarely will a person with high levels of BP experience a severe headache; some headaches are experienced in the morning and often subside on arising. It should be emphasized that it is impossible for most individuals to know whether their BP is elevated by the way they feel (see Question 9).

> *Primary hypertension very rarely causes symptoms or signs that warn individuals about their elevated blood pressure. As a consequence, disease complications from hypertension may occur before the blood pressure elevation is recognized—hence the name "the silent killer."*

Primary hypertension accounts for elevated BP in approximately 95 percent of the 72 million Americans who have hypertension. It is more correct to consider high BP to be an abnormal condition of the regulation of the circulation rather than a specific disease, as the causes of this form of hypertension remain unknown. Although genetic and environmental factors (especially obesity and excess sodium consumption) are often directly related to the development of hypertension, exactly how each factor promotes hypertension remains unclear (see Questions 6, 13, 33).

With secondary types of hypertension, a specific disease causes the elevated BP (See Question 38). Symptoms, signs, and certain biochemical abnormalities are frequently present with this type of hypertension, and this can permit a physician to make the diagnosis at a relatively early stage of the disease.

Because primary hypertension may remain silent for many years and lead to serious negative health outcomes, it is essential that everyone have their BP checked at least every one to two years. This minimal investment of time may yield maximal dividends — the protection and preservation of your health.

29 Can Thyroid Disease Be Causing My Hypertension, and What Are the Signs and Symptoms?

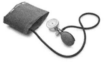

Both an overactive thyroid gland and an underactive thyroid gland can cause or aggravate hypertension. Nevertheless, abnormal thyroid function only rarely causes hypertension.

> In patients with hyperthyroidism, hypertension results from overproduction of the thyroid hormones, which stimulate the rate and pumping force of the heart, and usually cause typical signs and symptoms.

Approximately 20 to 30 percent of patients with an overactive thyroid gland (hyperthyroidism) have hypertension. This condition usually takes the form of mainly elevated systolic blood pressure; diastolic pressure is often decreased, but it may be increased by hyperthyroidism. Their hypertension results from overproduction of the thyroid hormones, which stimulate the rate and pumping force of the heart.

The typical signs and symptoms of hyperthyroidism are often readily apparent. The patient may have prominent eyes that give a scared or frightened appearance to the face, and may suffer from the following symptoms: nervousness, trembling, irritability, heat intolerance, excess sweating, palpitations (heart consciousness), diarrhea, insomnia, weight loss despite increased appetite, decreased menstruation, fatigue, and a variety of less-obvious signs and symptoms. The entire thyroid gland is usually enlarged but may have a discrete nodule or multiple nodules. In elderly patients, manifestations may be less obvious and perhaps include only cardiovascular symptoms such as angina (pain or pressure sensation in the chest and irregularity of the heart rhythm). The diagnosis is easily established by blood tests, which reveal excess concentrations of the thyroid hormones. With appropriate treatment, the hypertension usually disappears or returns to its previous level.

A small percentage of the total hypertensive population has been reported to have an underactive thyroid gland, a condition known as hypothyroidism. In individuals with hypothyroidism and hypertension, both systolic and diastolic pressures are elevated, which appears to result from the activation of the sympathetic nervous system and constriction of arterioles. These patients usually have a slow pulse and a decreased pumping force of the heart.

The signs and symptoms of hypothyroidism may include fatigue, lethargy, a slowing of intellectual function and physical activity, cold intolerance, a deepening of the voice and sometimes hoarseness, and dry skin and hair with some hair loss. The thyroid gland is usually not enlarged, although a goiter

> In patients with hypothyroidism, hypertension may result from activation of the sympathetic nervous system and constriction of arterioles. Deficiency of thyroid hormones may cause characteristic signs and symptoms.

(a very large thyroid) is sometimes readily evident. The diagnosis is easily confirmed by blood tests — the concentration of thyroid-stimulating hormone (TSH) is elevated in 95 percent of cases. Replacement of the deficient thyroid hormone usually returns the blood pressure to its previous level.

Because of the characteristic signs and symptoms of abnormal thyroid function and the availability of excellent blood tests for these conditions, it should not be difficult for the physician to determine whether thyroid malfunction is responsible for hypertension.

30 Can Hypertension Lead to Blindness?

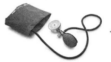

Only rarely does hypertension lead to blindness. The eyes are considered "target organs" of hypertension, because this condition can damage the small blood vessels in the retina (the membrane at the back of the eye that senses images formed by the lens, which are transmitted to the brain). Hypertension rarely leads to any of the various degrees of blindness (being "legally blind" implies very poor vision — unable to read, drive, or function without some help). When it does, the problem is usually temporary and eyesight improves with treatment of the hypertension. On the other hand, diabetes with or without hypertension often affects vision and can lead to blindness.

An ophthalmoscope can be employed to look through the lens at the small blood vessels in the retina, thereby enabling the physician to classify the severity of the hypertension, even if the eyesight is not affected. Evidence of hypertension as determined by the ophthalmoscope includes narrowing of retinal arterioles, hemorrhages, white patches (known as exudates) of various degrees, and swelling of the optic nerve, when the blood pressure remains very high for a prolonged period. Some of these changes in the retina and optic nerve may impair vision.

31 Can Hypertension Lead to Dialysis, and How Does Dialysis Work?

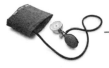

Hypertension is one of the leading causes of kidney failure and the need for dialysis. The kidneys are one of the "target organs" of hypertension. Untreated hypertension can lead to kidney failure with uremia (the accumulation of waste products and chemicals in the blood), which requires dialysis or transplantation. Next to diabetes, the most frequent cause for patients to undergo dialysis or a kidney transplant is hypertension. Effective treatment of high blood pressure will prevent this complication, especially when kidney function has not significantly deteriorated. Treatment, however, should begin before extensive damage to the kidneys occurs. Once such damage is present, treatment may slow the process, but it will not entirely prevent or reverse the problem.

> *Dialysis is a means of removing waste products and undesirable chemicals from the blood of patients with acute or chronic kidney failure.*

Dialysis is a means of removing waste products and undesirable chemicals from the blood of patients with acute or chronic kidney failure; chronic kidney failure is also known as end-stage renal (kidney) disease (ESRD). In hemodialysis, blood flows for about four hours from an artery through an external filter (which serves as an artificial kidney) and then back into a vein of the patient. The waste products and undesirable chemicals pass from the blood through a cellophane membrane into the dialyzing fluid, which is continually being discarded and replaced by a constant flow of fresh fluid. The "cleaned" blood returned to the body contains a much more normal composition than the blood before dialysis. Patients usually require dialysis several times each week.

32 Can Hypertension Cause Alzheimer's Disease or Dementia?

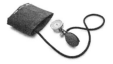

There is evidence that untreated hypertension is associated with midlife cognitive decline and vascular dementia; however, there is no definite evidence that hypertension can cause Alzheimer's disease. Patients who have never had hypertension can develop Alzheimer's disease, and treatment of hypertension does not seem to improve the condition. Multiple small strokes, however, sometimes result in a condition similar to Alzheimer's that is marked by progressive dementia (memory loss) called "multi-infarct dementia." This type of dementia is related to hypertension because hypertension is a risk factor for strokes. Unfortunately, although treatment of high blood pressure may prevent strokes, it does not improve multi-infarct dementia once it has occurred.

33 Is Hypertension Ever Familial, and Is There an Explanation for This Relationship?

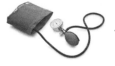

There is a strong familial link in primary hypertension, which accounts for 95 percent of all hypertension cases. If one parent has primary hypertension, 25 to 50 percent of their children will develop hypertension; if both parents have hypertension, the percentage of their children developing hypertension increases to almost 100 percent (see Questions 6, 13). The precise genetic defects that may explain this familial tendency to develop hypertension remain unclear, but multiple genes are involved and interact with one another and environmental factors. In addition, several hormonal systems and the sympathetic nervous system may play major roles in the development of hypertension.

> There is a strong familial link in primary hypertension, which accounts for 95 percent of all hypertension cases.

Notably, perhaps 60 percent of individuals with primary hypertension are salt sensitive; that is, their blood pressure becomes elevated when they consume excess amounts of table salt (sodium chloride). Some evidence indicates that the kidneys in salt-sensitive animals retain more sodium than the same organs in animals that are not salt sensitive. It seems likely that a similar condition may exist in salt-sensitive humans. It is noteworthy that the prevalence of hypertension is greater in African Americans and that this population is more likely to be salt sensitive than whites. Furthermore, African Americans usually develop hypertension at a younger age than whites, and their hypertension is more severe and accompanied by more serious health outcomes stemming from cardiovascular disease than hypertension in whites. Although these differences between African Americans and whites have genetic implications, the abnormalities remain undefined as yet.

A single gene abnormality is responsible for polycystic kidney disease, which frequently causes hypertension in family members and relatives. Some of these patients have high amounts of renin in the blood released from the cystic kidneys; the renin generates angiotensin, which can cause hypertension.

In addition, a number of very rare inherited conditions (accounting for about 0.2 percent of all hypertension cases) cause hypertension because of a single gene defect:

- In Liddle's syndrome a defect in the kidney tubules causes too much retention of sodium and water.

- In glucocorticoid remedial aldosteronism (GRA) the hypertension results from too much aldosterone hormone being produced by the adrenal glands, leading to excess retention of sodium and water.

- In congenital adrenal hyperplasia (an enlargement of the adrenal glands), the hypertension results from an enzyme defect that leads to the production of a steroid that causes retention of excess sodium and water.

In the above mentioned rare conditions, sodium and water retention lead to expansion of the blood volume, which then increases the pumping force of the heart, causing hypertension (see Question 38).

Another rare form of familial hypertension results from tumors of the adrenal glands that secrete epinephrine and norepinephrine. This can increase the pumping force of the heart and cause constriction of arterioles, thereby raising blood pressure. These rare familial tumors, which occur with other endocrine tumors and abnormalities, are known as multiple endocrine neoplasia (MEN) syndromes. A genetic abnormality has been detected in most patients with these tumors, and they can occur in many family members and their relatives (see Question 35).

Finally, preeclampsia has a hereditary tendency. This condition has been reported in 25 percent of daughters and granddaughters of patients who have experienced preeclampsia. As yet, the explanation for preeclampsia's development and familial occurrence remains unknown.

34. What Is the Story on Salt? How Much Can I Use? What about Salt Substitutes?

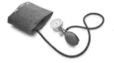

Table salt contains 40 percent sodium and 60 percent chloride, and sodium plays a role in causing high blood pressure (BP) in 50 to 60 percent of people with hypertension. For example, adequate dietary sodium restriction and increased sodium elimination caused by diuretics (taking "water pills") can significantly lower BP in some people with hypertension. In addition, human population studies and clinical trials provide data demonstrating a strong relationship between the amount of salt eaten and hypertension. Finally, in certain experimental animal models, including apes, unequivocal evidence shows that excess salt (sodium chloride) consumption causes hypertension.

> *Salt plays a role in causing high blood pressure in 50 to 60 percent of all people with hypertension.*

In the hypertensive population, roughly 75 percent of African Americans and 60 percent of white people are salt sensitive. Salt sensitivity is also particularly common in obese individuals, diabetics, and people older than sixty-five. The only way to determine whether you are sensitive to salt is to see whether going from a very low-salt to a very high-salt diet significantly increases your BP, or to see if going from a high-salt to a low-salt diet lowers your BP. Excess salt consumption appears to decrease blood flow and salt excretion by the kidneys of salt-sensitive animals and people, whereas the kidneys of normal animals and individuals increase their blood flow and excretion of salt under the same circumstances. Excess amounts of salt cause constriction of arterioles in salt-sensitive individuals, thereby increasing BP; the reason for this arterial constriction remains unknown.

Although the greater occurrence and severity of hypertension in African Americans versus whites remains unexplained, it has been suggested that the kidneys of African Americans are more likely to retain salt than are the kidneys of white individuals (see Question 26). Some African Americans may consume less potassium than whites, which may explain why they have more severe hypertension than whites; potassium appears to oppose the accumulation of sodium in the body and can dilate arteries and decrease BP. In addition, a deficiency of calcium or magnesium may also contribute to elevated BP. The exact interactions among sodium, potassium, calcium, and magnesium in BP regulation remain to be elucidated (see Question 98).

Americans consume roughly twenty times the amount of salt a person requires for normal body function. More than 75 percent of ingested salt comes from processed food (that is, food prepared by companies for public consumption); about 12 percent comes from natural, unprocessed food; and about 11 percent is added in the household. People with hypertension should read the labels on processed foods to become familiar with the amounts of sodium they are consuming. Foods with more than 400 mg of sodium per portion should be avoided.

The National High Blood Pressure Education Program (a former coalition of about forty-five national professional and federal agencies, of which the National Hypertension Association and the American Society of Hypertension were members) and the American Heart Association recommend a daily dietary intake of no more than 6 grams (g) of salt (sodium chloride); this is equivalent to 2,400 mg of sodium. The average American now consumes about twice this amount, much more than is required for proper nutrition. The Institute of Medicine recommends that for the prevention of hypertension, no more than 1,500 mg of sodium be consumed a day. Reduction of sodium intake to this level appears to be both safe and achievable, and it might reduce the number of people developing hypertension and decrease the yearly mortality rate from stroke and heart attack. Currently, it is recommended that sodium intake for African Americans, people with hypertension and/or impaired kidney function, and adults over forty years old be limited to 1,500 mg of sodium per day, whereas sodium intake for other adults be limited to 2,300 mg per day. Reducing dietary sodium will enhance the effectiveness of most antihypertensive drugs and may eliminate the need of medication in some hypertensives.

> *The National High Blood Pressure Education Program and the American Heart Association recommend a daily intake of no more than 6 g of salt.*

Limiting sodium intake should be combined with other types of healthful lifestyle changes, if indicated, such as weight reduction, smoking cessation, limiting consumption of alcohol, and getting adequate exercise. A diet low in saturated fats and cholesterol (which is mainly found in animal tissues and dairy products) but high in fiber and fruits and vegetables (which will increase potassium intake) is also recommended. Fresh foods have very little sodium, and the addition of pepper, spices, herbs, lemon, onion, garlic, vinegar, table wine, horseradish, unsalted mustard or catsup, and Worcestershire sauce (with low sodium) can add wonderful flavor to your food and help you kick the salt habit.

Some common foods high in sodium are listed in Table 2. Beware of particularly high sources of sodium. These items include

Table 2. Examples of Common Foods, Some with High Sodium Levels

Food	Amount	Sodium (mg)
American cheese, processed	1 oz	405
Bouillon, canned	1 cup	782
Cheddar or Colby cheese, low sodium	1 oz	6
Cream cheese	1 oz	84
Frankfurter, beef	1 serving	461
Frozen dinner, fried chicken meal, with mashed potatoes and corn	1 serving	1,500
Frozen dinner, meat loaf with mashed potatoes and carrots	1 serving	1,943
Italian sausage	1 link	665
Juice, tomato, canned	½ cup	438
Meat, canned	1 oz	394
Olives, canned	3	120
Pickles, dill	1 spear	384
Pizza, cheese	1 slice	336
Pot pie, beef	1 serving	736
Pot pie, turkey	1 serving	1,390
Salad dressing, Thousand Island	1 tbsp	109
Soup, chicken noodle, canned	1 cup	849
Soup, lentil with ham, canned	1 cup	1,319
Soy sauce	1 tbsp	1,005
Spaghetti and meatballs, canned	1 cup	940
Swiss cheese	1 oz	73

(Source: U.S. Department of Agriculture, Agricultural Research Service. 1999. USDA Nutrient Database for Standard Reference, Release 13. Nutrient Data Laboratory home page, http://www.nal.usda.gov/fnic/foodcomp.)

anchovies, bacon, baking powder/soda, bouillon, bologna and other smoked meats, bread, butter, canned soups and vegetables, catsup, cheese, cocoa mix, dill pickles, English muffins, frankfurters, ham, nuts, pancake mix, popcorn, pretzels, salted potato chips, sardines, sauerkraut, tomato juice, tuna in oil, and waffles.

Salt substitutes and "lite salt" should not be used without the recommendation of a physician. Many substitutes contain potassium chloride, which may be hazardous to those with impaired kidney function or those taking certain antihypertensive drugs that cause potassium retention. Evidence indicates that potassium may produce a beneficial effect by replacing sodium in cells and eliminating sodium in the urine, thereby lowering blood pressure. We also caution against the use of salt tablets to counteract salt and water loss, even with excess sweating in hot weather, unless recommended by a physician. It is noteworthy that sea salt contains as much sodium as table salt. For individuals who are particularly fond of salt, it is comforting to note that limiting salt in your diet will eventually decrease your desire for this compound and may actually make food taste better without it. So *bon appetit*!

35 Is My Nervousness Caused by Too Much Epinephrine, and Can This Condition Elevate My Blood Pressure?

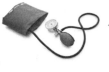

If you feel nervous, anxious, tense, apprehensive, or fearful, and you experience a rapid and pounding heartbeat with elevated blood pressure and sometimes with sweating, it is reasonable to wonder whether too much epinephrine is present in your blood. Although an overactive sympathetic nervous system may partly explain your emotional disturbance, this is not ordinarily accompanied by any increase in the circulation of either epinephrine (released from the adrenal gland) or norepinephrine (released from sympathetic nerves). On the other hand, when strenuous exercise or emotional anxiety activates the "fight-or-flight" response, a modest increase of these hormones in the blood can occur and may be associated with transitory hypertension and a rapid heart rate.

Nevertheless, a rare but treacherous and potentially lethal tumor known as a pheochromocytoma (fe-o-kro´-mo-si-to´-mah) can cause enormous increases of epinephrine and norepinephrine in the blood. This condition produces either sustained or periodic elevations of blood pressure as well as a rapid heart rate (see Questions 33, 36, 38). Approximately 90 percent of such tumors arise in the adrenal glands, which are located on the top of each kidney. In some patients they arise elsewhere in the abdomen (including the urinary bladder) and on rare occasions in the chest or neck. Roughly 10 percent of pheochromocytomas are familial (occurring in the same family or in relatives), and these cases may be associated with cancers of the thyroid gland and tumors of the parathyroid glands. Occasionally patients with this familial disease will have nodules on the lips and tongue and other manifestations. Although pheochromocytoma is a rare cause of hypertension — occurring perhaps only once in every two thousand hypertensive patients with both systolic and diastolic hypertension — it requires special vigilance by the physician to detect this "needle in the haystack" so that it can be promptly removed.

> *An overactive sympathetic nervous system is not ordinarily accompanied by any increase in the blood of either adrenaline or noradrenaline. On the other hand, a modest increase of these hormones in the blood can occur with the "fight-or-flight" response and be associated with transitory hypertension and a rapid heart rate.*

Most commonly, people with a pheochromocytoma complain of headaches, sweating for no apparent reason, and a rapid heart rate with palpitations (the feeling that the heart is pounding stronger than usual). There is often extreme pallor (paleness) of the face (rarely flushing), sometimes a tremor of the hands, and occasionally a marked fear of impending death. Abdominal and chest pain; weight loss; visual disturbances; numbness, tingling, and pain in the extremities; and constipation or diarrhea may be experienced by some patients. Rarely, fever may occur and suggest an infection.

Most symptoms and signs occur repeatedly in a dramatic and explosive manner without any warning and may be experienced several times each day or only once every few months. Because of the explosive nature of these attacks, pheochromocytoma has been described as a pharmacologic time bomb or a volcano that erupts periodically. These periodic attacks usually last about fifteen minutes but may sometimes persist for hours, leaving the individual exhausted after the attack subsides. The blood pressure is often markedly elevated during events but may remain normal between them. If these hormones are released into the blood continuously, then the blood pressure may remain persistently elevated. In such cases, symptoms and signs may be experienced chronically but less severely than when attacks occur periodically. Attacks may sometimes be precipitated by a change in posture, exercise, anxiety, the ingestion of certain foods or alcoholic beverages, the consumption of fruit juice, hyperventilation, straining, smoking, pressure in the area of the tumor, sexual intercourse, the administration of certain drugs, operative manipulation, and childbirth. If the tumor is located in the urinary bladder, attacks may be precipitated by bladder distension or urination.

Because approximately 95 percent of patients with pheochromocytoma are symptomatic, a detailed history and physical examination can prove valuable in determining which patients with sustained or intermittent hypertension should be screened for this tumor. All symptomatic patients with sustained or labile (fluctuating) hypertension should be screened by measuring the levels of these hormones (or their metabolites), as pheochromocytomas secrete these substances into either the urine or blood. Once the diagnosis has been established, the tumor must be located by radiological techniques (such as a computerized axial tomography, or CAT, scan), magnetic resonance imaging (MRI), or use of a radiolabled substance that seeks out the tumor.

If you have any of the possible manifestations of pheochromocytoma, you should mention them to your physician. Only very rarely are patients with signs and symptoms of excess epinephrine and norepinephrine harboring a pheochromocytoma, but in such cases, the proper diagnosis must be either confirmed or excluded so as to avoid the serious, and perhaps lethal, consequences of an unrecognized tumor.

36 What Causes a Sudden Elevation of Blood Pressure? Should Labile (Fluctuating) Blood Pressure Be Treated in Normal and Hypertensive People?

Blood pressure (BP) fluctuates remarkably in both normal individuals and those with hypertension. Furthermore, this fluctuation, or lability, of BP varies among different people and is influenced by many factors.

Stimulation of the nervous system can cause the blood vessels to constrict and increase the pumping force of the heart, which in turn elevates BP (see Question 14). This increase in nervous system activity and BP is greater in the morning and when a person first arises. Consequently, BP is usually higher in the morning than in the evening and is lowest during sleep. During routine daily activities, however, the BP can become rapidly elevated to a significant degree. For example, physical activity will increase systolic BP, with the effect especially pronounced during strenuous aerobic exercise. Anaerobic exercise such as very heavy weight lifting can, on occasion, increase systolic BP to as high as 300 mm Hg! This type of exercise should be avoided unless BP is normal.

In addition, the anxiety of having one's BP taken by the doctor may cause a significant BP elevation in about 20 percent of people who do not have hypertension. This is called "white-coat" hypertension (see Question 14). Likewise, the fear and anger that may occur during a hostile encounter or the fright of a dangerous or threatening experience (for example, almost being struck by a car) can powerfully stimulate the nervous system and produce a marked rise in BP, accompanied by a rapid heartbeat and a pounding in the chest. This reaction, due to the activation of the sympathetic nerves and the release of epinephrine, was termed the "fight-or-flight" response by the late physiologist Walter Canon.

Some illicit drugs — especially cocaine, amphetamines, and some herbal remedies such as ephedra, which contains ephedrine — can cause marked transitory hypertension and can also, rarely, be lethal (see Question 71). Another rare cause of a marked elevation in blood pressure is a tumor that periodically releases hormones (epinephrine and norepinephrine) into the circulation (see Questions 35, 38). Usually this is associated with severe headaches, sweating, pallor (paleness), and pounding of the heart.

When the BP is monitored for twenty-four hours, the marked variability in normal people is very evident. Many factors — caffeine, nicotine from cigarette smoking, an evening of excessive alcohol consumption — can temporarily elevate BP. The periodic stress encountered in one's job or associated with family and social problems can also temporarily raise BP. Even mentally performing math problems or having a conversation may transiently elevate BP.

It is noteworthy, however, that BP fluctuations in response to the various stimuli mentioned previously are usually considerably greater in patients with untreated hypertension. These frequent fluctuations in BP are probably best explained by the fact that the arteries of hypertensive patients are already abnormally constricted and that any additional constriction caused by activation of the sympathetic nervous system results in an exaggerated BP elevation. The arteries of hypertensive subjects appear to be especially responsive to various stimuli that cause the constriction of blood vessels.

In summary, a large array of physical and emotional factors may cause fluctuations of BP throughout the day; some of these pressure elevations may be considerable even in normal individuals. No strong evidence exists to show that these temporary elevations are a health risk. In contrast, however, frequent fluctuations seen in patients with untreated hypertension may damage blood vessels and increase the risk of heart attack, stroke, and heart and kidney failure. For this reason, hypertensive patients should be treated so as to minimize or eliminate excessive BP fluctuations. If spontaneous marked elevations of BP occur periodically, especially if accompanied by headaches, sweating, pounding of the heart, and pallor (paleness), the diagnosis of a tumor that secretes epinephrinelike hormones should be considered and the diagnosis confirmed or eliminated (see Question 35).

> Temporary elevations of blood pressure are not a health risk, but frequent fluctuations seen in some patients with untreated hypertension may damage blood vessels and increase the risk of heart attack, stroke, and heart and kidney failure.

37 What Is Isolated Systolic Hypertension, and Should It Be Treated?

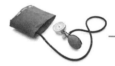

The term *isolated systolic hypertension* (ISH) describes the situation in which systolic blood pressure (BP) is elevated, but diastolic BP is less than 90 mm Hg. For example, a BP of 180/80 mm Hg would be considered ISH. This condition is especially common in elderly patients (usually older that fifty-five years) and is associated with an increased risk of stroke, heart failure, and heart attacks. ISH in elderly patients is usually a reflection of widespread "hardening" of the large arteries (arteriosclerosis). ISH is uncommon in patients younger than forty years of age. When it occurs in these individuals, it usually reflects an

> In isolated systolic hypertension, systolic blood pressure is elevated, but diastolic blood pressure is normal.

overactive heart that pumps increased amounts of blood; it is often a forerunner of systolic and diastolic hypertension later in life.

People with elevated systolic BP should always be treated. For many years the decision to treat elevated systolic BP was a source of concern and debate among physicians. We now know that we can reduce BP in people with this type of hypertension and that lowering the systolic BP is beneficial and not harmful as was once feared. In fact, the benefits of treating ISH are even greater and more immediately realized than the benefits of treating systolic and diastolic hypertension in younger patients. Studies have shown a remarkable 50 percent decrease in heart failure in ISH patients who received treatment as compared with those who received a sugar pill (a placebo [see Question 74]); the former group also saw significant reductions in heart attacks and strokes, and mortality from any cause was reduced significantly.

38 What Are the Causes of Secondary Hypertension, and How Can You Identify Them?

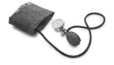

Only some 5 percent of the 72 million hypertensive individuals in the United States have an identifiable cause of their elevated blood pressure, and they are thus considered to have what is called secondary hypertension. The other 95 percent of patients have primary hypertension, in which the precise cause of the condition remains unknown. The good news is that secondary hypertension can sometimes be cured with surgery or successfully treated with medication, and primary hypertension can be controlled with lifestyle changes and/or medication.

The following findings suggest the presence of secondary hypertension: the sudden onset of hypertension in childhood or after the age of fifty years, especially if it is severe and accompanied by unusual symptoms, if it is resistant to treatment with medication, if certain abnormalities are found on physical examination, and if no family history of hypertension exists. A large number of conditions can cause secondary hypertension, some of which are listed in Table 3. It is beyond the scope of this book to discuss all of the underlying causes of such hypertension and the means of diagnosing each condition, so only the most frequent causes of secondary hypertension will be mentioned here and in the text following the table.

Table 3. Major Secondary Causes of Hypertension

Diagnosis	Conditions Responsible for Secondary Hypertension
Kidney damage (nephropathy) and/or impaired function	a. Diseases involving kidney tissue (not curable) Glomerulonephritis (acute or chronic inflammation) Diabetic nephropathy Polycystic kidney disease Lupus nephropathy Drug-induced nephropathy Injury-induced kidney damage b. Narrowing of artery or arteries to kidneys (sometimes curable) Atherosclerotic Fibromuscular disease c. Liddle's Syndrome (treatable but not curable)
Endocrine abnormality	a. Adrenal tumors or overactivity of adrenal glands Aldosteronoma or excess aldosterone secretion (curable or treatable) Familial enzyme abnormalities causing release of excess aldosterone (not curable) Pheochromocytoma (usually curable) Cushing's syndrome or disease (sometimes curable) b. Overactive thyroid gland (curable) Underactive thyroid gland (treatable) c. Oral contraceptives (curable) d. Acromegaly—overactive pituitary gland (curable) e. Overactive parathyroid glands (sometimes curable)
Preeclampsia (toxemia of pregnancy) or eclampsia	Occurs in third trimester of pregnancy (curable)

(cont'd.)

Table 3. Major Secondary Causes of Hypertension (cont'd.)

Diagnosis	Conditions Responsible for Secondary Hypertension	
Nervous system disorders or diseases	a. Increased pressure on the brain b. Brain tumors c. Convulsive seizures d. Quadriplegia from spinal cord injury e. Infections f. Lead or mercury poisoning	sometimes curable
Sleep apnea	It is not clear whether treatment cures hypertension	

Note: The diagnoses listed in this table account for only 5 percent of all people with hypertension. You should discuss these secondary causes of hypertension with your physician to obtain more detailed information regarding treatment and curability.

Kidney damage and impaired function account for most secondary forms of hypertension. Various types of nephritis (inflammation) or damage to kidney tissue (e.g., diabetic nephropathy) can usually be easily detected by increased amounts of protein and blood cells in the urine and sometimes by retention of chemicals in the blood that are ordinarily eliminated by normal kidneys. Polycystic kidneys can usually be felt in the abdomen because of significant enlargement; the presence of these enlarged kidneys with cysts is easily demonstrated by imaging studies (such as ultrasound or X rays of the kidneys). Because polycystic kidney disease is due to a genetic defect, it often affects other family members in addition to the patient (see Question 33).

A narrowing (stenosis) of an artery to one or both kidneys can cause significant ischemia (impaired blood supply) to kidney tissue, thereby stimulating release of an enzyme called renin. Renin release generates angiotensin, a hormone that causes constriction of arterioles and thus raises blood pressure. Stenosis of an artery to the kidney is the most common cause of curable secondary hypertension, but it accounts for less than 1 percent of the hypertensive population. The stenosis usually results from atherosclerosis accompanied by cholesterol plaque formation and partial obstruction of blood flow to the kidney. This obstruction usually occurs in the elderly. The obstruction of kidney arteries may also result from fibromuscular dysplasia, an overgrowth of smooth muscle cells in the walls of these arteries. This condition is most often seen in young women, especially those who smoke cigarettes. There is also a rare form of abnormality of the arteries in the kidneys that can cause hypertension, particularly in women from East Asia, called Takayasu's disease.

The sudden onset of hypertension in the elderly or young women (especially those who have been cigarette smokers) with the presence of a certain type of murmur (bruit) in the abdomen near the kidneys suggests stenosis (narrowing or constriction) of a kidney artery. The physician must then determine whether the stenosis is responsible for the hypertension. Certain imaging techniques can reveal a constriction of the artery, accompanied by a reduced blood flow and an increased hormone level that constricts arteries and elevates blood pressure.

Liddle's syndrome is a very rare genetic abnormality of the kidney that causes excess sodium retention, which in turn expands blood volume and causes hypertension. It can be identified through blood tests (see Question 33).

After kidney-related conditions, endocrine-related defects (particularly tumors of the adrenal gland) are the next most common cause of secondary hypertension. *Aldosteronomas* are tumors that occur in the outer portion of the adrenal gland. They secrete excess amounts of aldosterone, a hormone that retains sodium, which in turn significantly expands blood volume and promotes an increase in the pumping force of the heart, constriction of arterioles, and hypertension. These types of tumors may be responsible for the hypertension in less than 1 percent of all patients. Tests identify this condition by detecting increased amounts of aldosterone in the blood and urine as well as low levels of potassium and renin in the blood. Patients may complain of weakness, headaches, and increased urination. Excess aldosterone may also result from an overgrowth and overactivity of the cells that produce aldosterone in the adrenal gland. These conditions may be identified by a CAT scan of the adrenal glands but, more often, detection usually requires obtaining blood from the veins draining the adrenal glands to determine which gland is responsible. In addition, several rare, inherited abnormalities of enzymes in the adrenal gland can lead to excess production of aldosterone or deoxycorticosterone (a similar hormone); extra amounts of these hormones cause retention of sodium, increase blood volume, and result in hypertension (see Question 33).

Pheochromocytomas account for about 0.05 percent of cases of hypertension. Most such tumors (90 percent) occur in the inner portion of the adrenal gland, although in some patients they may arise elsewhere in the abdomen and the pelvis, including in the urinary bladder and in the area where the aorta divides to supply blood to the legs. Occasionally pheochromocytomas occur in the region of the heart and in the back portion of the chest near the spine; on rare occasions they occur in the neck. These tumors usually secrete epinephrine and norepinephrine, both of which increase the pumping force of the heart, constrict most arterioles, and elevate blood pressure (see Question 35). About 50 percent of these tumors cause sustained hypertension, whereas 45 percent cause only periodic hypertension — often with dramatic manifestations such as severe headaches, palpitations (heart consciousness), excess sweating, pallor (paleness), and severe anxiety. A small percentage of these tumors do not cause hypertension. Thirty percent are inherited and occur in members of a family and relatives.

Cushing's syndrome and *Cushing's disease* result when the adrenal glands secrete excessive amounts of the hormone cortisol into the blood. The syndrome (a group of manifestations) can result from a tumor of the pituitary gland (Cushing's disease), tumors of the adrenal glands, and, rarely, other tumors. The syndrome is frequently caused by the administration of corticosteroids (for example, prednisone) as a treatment for various diseases. Cortisol often causes hypertension and produces a very characteristic body appearance that includes abdominal obesity, excess body hair, a round "moon" face, purple streaks on the abdomen, and a protuberance of fatty tissue in the back of the neck called a "buffalo hump." Cushing's syndrome is more frequently observed in women and is often accompanied by emotional disturbances, lack of menstrual periods, fatigue, and easy bruising. Blood tests, CAT scans of the adrenal glands, and an MRI scan of the pituitary gland can usually pinpoint whether this endocrine condition is due to an adrenal or pituitary abnormality.

An overactive thyroid gland (resulting in increased thyroid hormones) usually elevates systolic blood pressure but lowers diastolic blood pressure; in some patients, diastolic pressure may also be elevated. An enlarged thyroid gland, prominent eyes, excessive inappropriate sweating, heat intolerance, diarrhea, weight loss, nervousness, a tremor of the hands, and rapid heartbeat frequently occur in individuals with hyperthyroidism. The increased rate and pumping force of the heart caused by excessive amounts of thyroid hormone in the circulation is mainly responsible for the elevated blood pressure. The diagnosis is easily established through thyroid function tests (see Question 29).

An underactive thyroid gland (resulting in decreased thyroid hormone) is associated with a slowing of the heart rate and a decrease in the pumping force of the heart; the arterioles constrict so as to maintain adequate circulation to the tissues, which increases blood pressure (especially the diastolic pressure). A deficiency of thyroid hormone in children can result in short stature, coarse features, impaired mental development, etc.; an enlarged thyroid gland (goiter) is usually present. In adults, symptoms of hypothyroidism may be mistakenly attributed to aging or a disease involving the nervous system. Patients often complain of fatigue, lethargy, cold intolerance, constipation, weight gain, a slowing of intellectual and muscle activity, loss of hair, dry skin, and a hoarse voice. The thyroid gland is usually not enlarged unless a goiter is present. Blood testing of thyroid activity will establish the diagnosis (see Question 29).

The *oral contraceptives* used today rarely cause hypertension, given their lower concentrations of estrogen and progesterone. Nevertheless, if hypertension occurs as a result of using the "pill," it may be severe. In most women who experience this problem, blood pressure will return to normal levels two or three months after discontinuing use of the pill. The reasons why hypertension develops are unclear, although sodium retention, blood volume expansion, and an increase in the pumping force of the heart may play a role.

Acromegaly results from the presence of excess growth hormone. This condition is characterized by gigantism (tall stature), with enlarged hands, feet, and jaw and coarsening of the facial features. Visual defects may arise if a pituitary tumor (usually the cause of excess growth hormone production) places pressure on the nerves to the eyes. Hypertension occurs in about 50 percent of acromegalics and may be related to sodium retention, an expanded blood volume with an increase in the pumping force of the heart, and constriction of arterioles. The diagnosis is made by the presence of the characteristic body changes and assessing growth hormone elevations in the blood when measured under appropriate circumstances. An MRI of the brain can usually identify a pituitary tumor that is responsible for acromegaly.

Overactive parathyroid glands in the neck cause the release of excess amounts of parathyroid hormone and an increased concentration of calcium in the blood, which is occasionally accompanied by hypertension. Patients usually have no symptoms, but excess urination and water drinking, along with constipation, kidney stones, peptic ulcer, and loss of calcium from the bones may occur. Diagnosis can be made by identifying increased parathyroid hormone and increased calcium concentrations in the blood.

Some drugs, drinks, and food may elevate blood pressure (see Table 3 on page 61). Some of these substances cause hypertension by activating the sympathetic nervous system, which causes the constriction of arterioles and hypertension. Others on the list promote the retention of sodium with expansion of blood volume and an increase in the pumping force of the heart, as well as an increase in the constriction of arterioles.

Coarctation is an inherited, congenital constriction of the aorta that usually occurs in the chest just beyond the blood vessels carrying blood to the arms. In this condition, blood pressure is elevated in the arms and upper portion of the body but is decreased in the portion of the body below the constriction. The cause of the hypertension in the upper body appears to be mainly the result of an obstruction of blood flow caused by the constriction; however, the constriction of arterioles throughout the body may result from increased activity of the sympathetic nerves and an elevated level of angiotensin in the blood. Frequently a murmur can be heard near the coarctation. The presence of elevated pressure in the arms, low pressure in the legs, and characteristic imaging studies establish the diagnosis (see Question 13).

In pregnant women, preeclampsia should be suspected if hypertension, a significant increase of protein (albumin) in the urine, and fluid retention (manifested by rapid excessive weight gain and swelling of the ankles) occur after the twentieth week of pregnancy (see Question 58). The cause of preeclampsia (toxemia of pregnancy) remains unknown. The blood pressure of patients with this condition should be carefully controlled. Preeclampsia may occasionally be followed by *eclampsia* — a condition characterized by severe hypertension and sometimes swelling of the brain and convulsions. Eclampsia proves fatal in 18 percent of cases. Preeclampsia can be cured and eclampsia can be prevented by delivery of the fetus. Only very rarely does it occur after delivery.

A number of nervous-system disorders or diseases may activate the sympathetic nervous system and cause the constriction of arteries and hypertension. MRI studies of the brain may be helpful in demonstrating brain abnormalities. Heavy metal poisoning can be demonstrated by elevated levels of the metals in the blood.

Sleep apnea usually occurs in middle-aged adults (2 percent of women and 4 percent of men); hypertension affects more than 50 percent of these individuals (see Question 61). Most sleep apnea results from airway obstruction, which is most commonly found in individuals with upper-body obesity. Loud snoring and episodes of gasping nearly always occur in people with sleep apnea, and daytime drowsiness is common. An overnight sleep study can identify sleep apnea.

39 How Can I Tell if My Hypertension Is Due to a Diseased or Damaged Kidney?

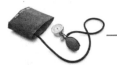

> If evidence of a kidney abnormality existed before the high blood pressure became a recognized issue, then this kidney defect likely preceded the high blood pressure and, therefore, may have caused it. If no evidence of kidney disease existed before high blood pressure affected the patient for several years, then the kidney damage likely resulted from the hypertension.

Because the kidney is a target organ of hypertension and can also cause hypertension, it is sometimes difficult to tell whether kidney disease or damage caused the hypertension or resulted from it. If evidence of a kidney abnormality existed before the high blood pressure became a recognized issue, then this kidney defect likely preceded the high blood pressure and, therefore, may have caused it. On the other hand, if no evidence of kidney disease existed before high blood pressure affected the patient for several years, then the kidney damage likely resulted from the hypertension.

Examination of the patient's blood and urine can help determine whether a kidney problem is present. Sometimes X rays employing contrast dyes may be helpful; for example, a kidney angiogram (which reveals the caliber of the arteries to the kidneys and identifies any obstruction to blood flow) or an MRI angiogram (which may reveal abnormalities of the arteries to the kidneys without use of contrast material). These imaging studies permit identification of damage to the kidneys and/or to the arteries supplying them with blood. Other less-expensive imaging may reveal anatomical abnormalities (sonography) or functional abnormalities (Doppler study) of the kidneys.

In addition to being caused by a diseased or damaged kidney, hypertension can result from impaired blood supply to a kidney. This defect may promote the release of renin into the blood and the formation of angiotensin. The latter condition causes constriction of the arterioles, which in turn causes hypertension (see Question 38). Hypertension much more frequently results in strokes, heart attacks, and heart failure than kidney failure, and good control of high blood pressure can prevent or minimize kidney disease.

40 If I Stay Physically Fit and Maintain a Healthy Lifestyle, Can Hypertension Be Prevented or Controlled?

For some people, physical fitness can prevent hypertension or reduce elevated blood pressure (BP) to a normal level. Although not everyone will achieve their BP goal this way, it is certainly worth a try for those with stage 1 or prehypertension. Maintaining physical fitness — through regular aerobic exercise, proper weight control, the avoidance of excess alcohol consumption, and abstinence from smoking — is certainly

Maintaining physical fitness may sometimes prevent hypertension or reduce elevated blood pressure to a normal level.

extremely desirable. And, undoubtedly, adherence to such a program of physical fitness and consumption of a healthy diet can be excellent means of preventing hypertension and reducing BP. That being said, however, it is impossible to alter your genes, gender, age, and racial background. The genetic influence may be too powerful to enable physical fitness to prevent hypertension; furthermore, if BP is constantly relatively high — for example, systolic and diastolic pressures greater than 165 and 110 mm Hg, respectively — antihypertensive medication will almost certainly be required to normalize the pressure, and physical activity and fitness will help the medicines work even better.

Weight-loss is the most effective means of lowering BP without using antihypertensive drugs. Analysis of carefully controlled studies reveals that every 2.2 pounds (1 kilogram) of weight loss is accompanied by a fall in systolic and diastolic pressure of 1.6 and 1.3 mm Hg, respectively. In one study, a decrease of 23 pounds resulted in a reduction of systolic and diastolic pressure by 11 and 8 mm Hg, respectively.

In our discussion of weight loss (see Question 48), we emphasize the importance of reducing caloric intake mainly by reducing fat to no more than 30 percent of total calories consumed. Low-fat diets matched with an abundance of fresh fruits and vegetables and little red meat will aid in lowering BP. Increasing the expenditure of calories by undertaking regular aerobic exercise at least four or five times weekly is equally important for weight reduction. Finally, limiting sodium consumption to 2,400 mg of sodium per day (1,500 mg is better) and restricting alcohol consumption to no more than one or two drinks of wine, beer, or spirits per day will help prevent BP from rising (see Question 34).

These lifestyle-change recommendations are discussed elsewhere in this book (see Questions 24, 34, 46, 47, 49, 51, 88, 89). If these changes are made and physical fitness is maintained, a significant number of individuals with stage 1 hypertension may be able to reduce their BP to a normal range; furthermore, the development of hypertension may be prevented in people who restrict their sodium consumption to no more than 2,400 mg per day. If lifestyle changes do not normalize BP after several months, antihypertensive drugs are added to the therapy. Appropriate lifestyle changes will also lessen the amount of antihypertensive medication required to control BP.

41 What Are Some of the Prescription, Over-the-Counter, and Illicit Drugs That Can Elevate Blood Pressure? What about Cold Medications?

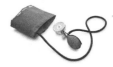

It is important for patients with hypertension and even individuals without this condition to recognize that some over-the-counter (OTC) drugs may cause hypertension; furthermore, certain prescription drugs and some illicit drugs can also elevate blood pressure (BP). For this reason, it is important to ask your doctor about any drug effects or interactions that could affect your BP or prove harmful.

> Drugs that can elevate blood pressure include some steroid or sex hormones, narcotics, illicit drugs, some antidepressants, cyclosporine, erythropoietin, alcohol, disulfiram, appetite suppressants, phenylpropanolamine, nicotine, caffeine, licorice, nasal decongestants, salt-containing antacids, and nonsteroidal anti-inflammatory drugs.

Drugs that can elevate BP include some steroidal hormones, sex hormones, narcotics, illicit drugs, some antidepressants, cyclosporine (a drug used to suppress the immune system), erythropoietin and related drugs (used to correct anemias), alcohol, disulfiram (used in the treatment of alcoholics), appetite suppressants, phenylpropanolamine in diet pills, nicotine, caffeine, natural licorice or licorice added to chewing tobacco, nasal decongestants, antacids that contain high amounts of salt (sodium chloride), and nonsteroidal anti-inflammatory drugs (NSAIDs). Most of these drugs cause hypertension in one of two ways:

- They increase retention of sodium and water by the kidneys, which causes expansion of the blood volume and increases the pumping force of the heart.

- They increase the activity of the sympathetic nervous system, which leads to an acceleration of the heart rate and the constriction of arterioles.

All of these drug effects can, therefore, cause a rise in BP or even lead to hypertension.

Many cold medications, "sinus medications," and decongestants contain ephedrine, pseudoephedrine, phenylephrine, or phenylpropanolamine. These ingredients can constrict the arteries and arterioles in the membranes lining the nasal cavity, thereby decreasing secretions of mucus and relieving the symptoms of nasal congestion. Although inhaling massive doses of nasal decongestant medications may cause an increase in BP and a rapid heart rate because of their effect on arterioles throughout the body and stimulation of the heart, usually no significant rise in BP occurs with their use. However, some cold medications taken by mouth may significantly elevate BP, especially in hypertensives.

The NSAIDs are commonly used for arthritis treatment and for relief of all sorts of pain. They include aspirin, Advil, Motrin, Nuprin, Indocin, Orudis, Naprosyn, Clinoril, Ansaid, Feldene, Voltaren, Celebrex, and Aleve. NSAIDs can interfere with antihypertensive treatment, and a significant increase in blood pressure may occur when these drugs are used chronically. This hypertensive effect is reported to be less or insignificant with aspirin, Clinoril, Ansaid, and Celebrex.

The elevation of BP caused by NSAIDs results when these substances inhibit the action of hormones (prostaglandins) that cause the dilation of arterioles; this dilation is important for elimination of sodium and water. Older people, salt-sensitive people, people with impaired kidney function, and hypertensive people all have a greater risk of developing severe hypertension or aggravating preexisting hypertension with the chronic use of NSAIDs because of excess retention of sodium and water by the kidneys. In addition, NSAIDs can decrease the effectiveness of antihypertensive drugs and may occasionally cause an ulcer in the stomach or small intestine. Although Tylenol does not affect BP or cause ulcers, when it is taken in very large dosages (for long periods), it may sometimes damage the kidneys and impair kidney function, thereby causing hypertension.

It is important to talk with your doctor about potential drug interactions and to learn which drugs to avoid if you have hypertension.

42 What Are the Major Risk Factors for Developing Hypertension?

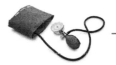

Observations made at periodic intervals in a large number of people, including children, suggest that the major risk factors for developing hypertension are a family history of hypertension in siblings or parents, excessive weight gain, a rapid resting pulse rate, and a diet high in salt (sodium chloride), especially in those who are salt sensitive.

43 What Are the Major Risk Factors for Cardiovascular and Kidney Disease, and How Can I Reduce the Chances of These Complications?

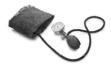

Risk factors for heart disease (including heart attack and heart failure), stroke, transient ischemic attack (TIA), and kidney disease include the following:

- hypertension
- diabetes mellitus
- cigarette smoking
- sedentary lifestyle
- obesity
- older age

- high LDL cholesterol ("bad" cholesterol)
- low HDL cholesterol ("good" cholesterol)
- high triglycerides (blood fat)
- family history of premature heart attack or stroke
- (for women) postmenopausal state

For any level of blood pressure, the presence of one or more of these risk factors will increase the likelihood of a heart attack, heart or kidney failure, or stroke. Thus, high blood pressure should be treated more intensively in individuals who have additional risk factors than in those who do not have such risk factors. The treatment of high cholesterol levels with the goal of lowering levels of LDLs and raising levels of HDL is equally important. Because age is also a risk factor, elderly patients should receive intensive treatment for high blood pressure and abnormal cholesterol levels, even if they do not have diabetes. Smoking cessation should be strongly urged, diabetes should be well controlled, and adequate exercise and a healthy diet should be included in your lifestyle (see Questions 44, 49, 51, 52, 62, 87, 89, 90, 95).

44 What Can I Do about Risk Factors if I Have Hypertension, and How Do They Affect Treatment?

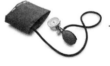

Some risk factors for hypertension (age, gender, genetic and racial background) obviously cannot be altered. In general, the risk of cardiovascular disease (heart attack, stroke, kidney and blood vessel damage) is greater in hypertensive men than in hypertensive women and greater in African Americans than in white Americans, especially as people age. Until age fifty, more men develop hypertension than women; however, after menopause, women are more likely to develop hypertension than men of the same age. Hypertension occurs more frequently in African Americans than in whites.

A history of premature cardiovascular disease in parents or siblings (that is, disease in men younger than fifty-five and in women younger than sixty-five years old) confers an additional risk for cardiovascular disease. If one parent has primary hypertension, 25 percent to 50 percent of their children are predisposed to develop the condition; if both parents have hypertension, almost 100 percent of their offspring will become hypertensive (see Questions 11, 13, 26, 33).

The good news is that environmental risk factors for hypertension can be modified or eliminated by doing the following:

- *Quitting smoking*, in addition to its many other benefits, will reduce the incidence of heart attacks and stroke and the damage to arteries caused by smoking (see Questions 51, 52).
- *Reducing weight* in individuals who are overweight will usually reduce elevated blood pressure (BP) and may help prevent development of hypertension (see Questions 47, 48, 49).
- *Curtailing excess salt consumption* can reduce and may help prevent hypertension, especially in salt-sensitive individuals (see Question 34).
- *Reducing elevated levels of LDL cholesterol* (low-density lipoprotein, the "bad" cholesterol) and *elevated levels of triglyceride fats, and increasing HDL cholesterol* (high-density lipoprotein, the "good" cholesterol) can reduce damage to arteries and prevent negative cardiovascular complications (see Questions 89, 90, 91).
- *Increasing exercise and avoiding a sedentary lifestyle* may improve the fitness of the heart, lower elevated BP, and aid in weight reduction (see Question 46).
- *Avoiding excessive alcohol consumption* may lower elevated BP and does reduce the number of calories obtained from the alcohol, which may be very helpful in weight reduction (see Question 24).
- *Maintaining a diet low in saturated fat and high in fiber, including liberal amounts of fruits and vegetables, which supply*

significant amounts of potassium, may not only lower BP, but may also reduce a person's incidence of stroke (see Question 49).

BP control is of crucial importance in reducing the occurrence of negative cardiovascular complications. Consequently, all the environmental factors mentioned above should be altered appropriately and medications utilized, if indicated. Finally, good control of diabetes is, of course, important in reducing the possibility of disease complications of diabetes; however, excellent BP control is even more important.

> Some risk factors for hypertension—age, gender, genetic, and racial background—obviously cannot be altered. The good news is that environmental risk factors can be modified or eliminated.

A useful strategy designed to improve the approach of treating hypertensive patients considers not only the level of BP elevation but also any major risk factors and evidence of damage to various organs and arteries of the body (listed below). Treatment is aimed at the following three risk groups and depends on the severity of BP elevation as well as the number of major risk factors and the amount of organ damage related to the hypertension.

Risk Group A

Risk group A includes patients with prehypertension or stage 1 or 2 hypertension (see Table 4) who do not have evidence of organ damage or other risk factors. Stage 1 patients may attempt to lower their BP with lifestyle changes and close monitoring of their

Table 4. Blood Pressure Classification

	Systolic (mm Hg)		Diastolic (mm Hg)
Optimal	Less than 120	and	Less than 80
Prehypertension	Range 120–139	or	Range 80–89
Stage 1	Range 140–159	or	Range 90–99
Stage 2	Greater than 160	or	Greater than 100

BP. If BP is not normalized within three to six months, antihypertensive drug therapy should be added. For patients with stage 2 hypertension, drug and lifestyle changes are indicated.

Risk Group B

Risk group B includes hypertensives who do not currently show evidence of organ damage but do have one or more of the major risk factors other than diabetes. This group accounts for the majority of hypertensive patients. If multiple risk factors are present, antihypertensive drugs and appropriate lifestyle modifications are indicated.

Risk Group C

Risk group C consists of hypertensive patients who have diabetes or evidence of organ damage. These individuals (and some people with high-normal BP as well as poor kidney function, heart failure, or diabetes) should be considered for prompt antihypertensive treatment plus appropriate lifestyle modifications.

Major Risk Factors

- cigarette smoking
- elevated levels of undesirable blood fats (LDL, triglycerides) and decreased levels of desirable blood fats (HDL)
- diabetes
- age greater than sixty years
- being a man or a postmenopausal woman
- a family history of premature cardiovascular disease (in men younger than fifty-five years old and in women younger than sixty-five)

Evidence of Organ Damage

- heart disease
  - enlargement of heart muscle of left ventricle (main pumping chamber)
  - chest pain (angina) or previous heart attack

- prior angioplasty (balloon dilation) or coronary bypass surgery
- heart failure
- stroke or transient ischemic attack (TIA; ministroke)
- kidney damage
- damage to arteries (especially in the legs)
- damage to the retinal portion of the eye

Of paramount importance for the most successful management of patients with various degrees of hypertension is a careful assessment of the major risk factors and evidence of cardiovascular disease and organ damage. This information will help the physician in selecting the most appropriate treatment for each patient.

45 What Is Target Organ Disease, and How Does Its Presence Influence Treatment?

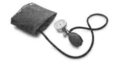

Target organ disease refers to disease in the organs that are most frequently damaged by high blood pressure — hence the term "target organs." The target organs of high blood pressure are the brain (strokes), the heart (heart attack and heart failure), the kidneys (kidney failure that may require dialysis), the eyes, and the arteries (arteriosclerosis or atherosclerosis). The presence of target organ damage is always a compelling reason to treat hypertension intensively so as to protect these organs and prevent further damage (see Question 44).

46 What Are the Benefits of Exercise, and Will It Lower My Blood Pressure?

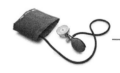

Exercise is essential for your health and physical fitness (see Questions 40, 43, 60). Unfortunately, in recent years, Americans have become increasingly passive spectators rather than active participants in physical activities. The advent of television, video games, and the Internet has greatly eroded the time spent exercising. Sadly, our children are particularly obsessed with television and computers. One study of ten-year-old American girls revealed a direct correlation between excess body fat and hours spent watching television. The increasing use of computers and similar devices will merely compound the problem, further eroding participation in physical activity and reducing physical fitness. Only 22 percent of adults get at least 30 minutes of exercise during most days.

Sedentary people ("couch potatoes") are more likely to develop hypertension and have heart attacks and strokes than people who are physically active. Furthermore, it has been demonstrated that regular, moderate aerobic exercise (that is, dynamic exercise that increases oxygen intake and increases activity of the heart, lungs, and muscles) may sometimes reduce systolic and diastolic blood pressure by about 10 and 8 mm Hg, respectively, in hypertensive subjects. It is noteworthy that moderate-intensity training appears to be just as effective as, if not better than, high-intensity exercise in providing many beneficial effects.

The benefits of regularly performing moderate aerobic exercise are many:

> *Sedentary people are more likely to develop hypertension and have heart attacks and strokes than people who are physically active. Regular, moderate aerobic exercise, on the other hand, may sometimes reduce both systolic and diastolic blood pressure in hypertensive subjects.*

- Such exercise may prevent or minimize damage to the coronary arteries of the heart and may improve heart function.

- Proper weight is more easily maintained.

- Muscle mass, strength, and agility are increased and preserved.

- Levels of the "good" blood cholesterol (HDL), which protects against hardening of the arteries, are increased, whereas levels of the "bad" cholesterol (LDL) and triglycerides (blood fats) are decreased.

• The risks of osteoporosis and diabetes are diminished.

• Emotional tension, anxiety, anger, and depression may be significantly alleviated.

It is especially important to choose enjoyable exercises; it is almost certain that a person will not stick with boring exercises for very long. Exercise intensity and duration should be increased gradually and then performed for thirty or more minutes most days of the week. Individuals over forty years old or anyone with any indication of heart or vascular disease should consult a physician before embarking on an exercise program.

Walking and jogging are particularly popular types of exercise that can be performed alone, with a few friends, or in large groups. Bicycling, tennis, paddle tennis, squash, volleyball, cross-country skiing, skating, roller-blading, golf, swimming, aerobic group exercise, or dancing are all excellent ways of getting the exercise needed to improve cardiovascular fitness and muscle strength. Exercise machines (such as the treadmill, rowing machine, stationary bicycle, stair climber, and the wide variety of dynamic muscle-building machines) are all excellent ways to work out and may be especially convenient; the opportunity to watch television, listen to music, or even read while using some of these machines can make the physical activity more enjoyable.*

Most of these moderate-intensity exercises pose little chance of injury, especially if a few minutes of muscle stretching — a warm-up period — precedes the exercise.

Although exercise will temporarily increase systolic pressure so as to increase blood flow to exercising muscle, systolic and dia-

---

* One word of caution regarding the use of a Walkman or mp3 player if jogging or roller-blading on a road: The possibility of being hit by a car is increased if your hearing is impaired. Jogging or roller-blading is safer if done in the direction of oncoming cars, so that you can see and avoid them.

stolic pressures may be lower for as long as several hours after the activity ends. No evidence has been found to suggest that regular, moderate-intensity exercise increases the risk of stroke or heart attack in hypertensive individuals. However, although lifting or "pressing" very heavy weights will build skeletal muscles, the straining required with isometrics (muscle contraction with little shorting but great increase in tone) should definitely be avoided. This type of activity can elevate both systolic and diastolic pressures; on rare occasions systolic pressures may reach 300 mm Hg or higher. Repetitive light weight lifting or exercises requiring the intermittent contraction and relaxation of muscles are permissible if not strenuous.

Moderately intense exercise for 30 minutes will burn up approximately 150 calories. If it is more desirable to perform two 15-minute or three 10-minute periods of exercise, the benefit and the total calories burned will be similar. Men burn up 10 to 20 percent more calories than women during exercise, probably due to men's greater muscle mass. One real benefit of physical activity is that, when combined with a reduced caloric intake, it can bring about significant weight loss and thereby further reduce blood pressure.

A good measure of fitness is your heart rate (pulse) and the length of time you can continue on a treadmill at different speeds. The maximum heart rate you should achieve during exercise decreases with age. The pulse rate at your wrist or in your neck, caused by exercising, should be recorded. With moderate exercise, this number should be roughly equivalent to 220 minus your age (the formula for maximum rate), multiplied by 70 percent (the recommended percent of the maximum rate that should be attained during moderate exercise). However, it is noteworthy that beta blockers can prevent the normal increase of heart rate with exercise. A physician should interpret the results of running on a treadmill, which is usually accompanied by an electrocardiogram (i.e., a stress test).

Most currently used antihypertensive medications do not interfere with the ability to exercise. Some drugs (beta blockers) that partially block the response of the heart to exercise will limit the pumping force of the heart and slow the pulse. Consequently, these drugs may reduce a person's capacity for strenuous physical activity.

Now that you know all of this, it should be obvious that the old adage "no pain, no gain" does not apply to exercise. Regularly performed, moderately intense exercise can be both very enjoyable and extremely beneficial to your health. So if there are no medical contraindications, start exercising regularly and discover the many ways to enjoy it!

47 Is It Important for Me to Lose Excess Weight if I Have Hypertension, and What Are the Reasons for and Risks of Being Overweight?

If you are moderately overweight, your chance of developing hypertension is three to six times greater than that of a healthy person with normal weight. If you are obese (that is, 20 percent or more above your ideal weight), your chance of developing hypertension may be as much as eight times greater than that of normal-weight individuals; hypertension affects approximately 50 percent of obese individuals (see Questions 40, 42, 46).

Obesity — defined as the excess accumulation of fat — is the most important environmental factor causing or aggravating hypertension. It may lead to retention of sodium and water, constrict arterioles, and force the heart to pump harder. Loss of even 10 pounds may significantly lower your elevated blood pressure. One study ....

> If you are moderately overweight, your chance of developing hypertension is three to six times greater than that of a healthy person with normal weight. If you are obese (that is, 20 percent or more above your ideal weight), your chance of developing hypertension may be as much as eight times greater than that of normal-weight individuals.

of obese hypertensive patients reported that the loss of 23 pounds caused average systolic and diastolic pressures to decline by 11 and 8 mm Hg, respectively. If you have prehypertension, weight loss may return your pressure to normal and prevent the need for medication. In addition, weight loss may reduce the amount of antihypertensive medication that is required. Weight reduction can also lower your total cholesterol (particularly your low-density lipoprotein [LDL] cholesterol, which is the "bad" cholesterol), and decrease your risk of developing atherosclerosis (hardening of the arteries) or diabetes or of having a heart attack or stroke.

Another reason for losing excess weight is that obesity predisposes an individual to the development of gallstones, degenerative arthritis, varicose veins and blood clots, toxemia of pregnancy, hernias, and many cancers. Furthermore, in obese people, surgery is technically more difficult and complications of surgery are more frequent, wounds don't heal as fast, and infections are more common. These conditions usually account for the relatively high premature death rate associated with significant obesity. The more you weigh, the greater the risks.

Excess fat is a national health problem in the United States. Based on measurements of body mass index (BMI), approximately 65 percent of all Americans are overweight and 32 percent are obese (20 percent or more above ideal weight). Americans are fatter than people in other large developed nations. Although the percentage of people who are overweight has increased slightly in the last forty years, the percentage of those who are obese has doubled! A simple way to determine ideal weight is the following:

- For men, use 106 pounds for the first 5 feet, then add 6 pounds for each additional inch of height.

- For women, use 100 pounds for the first 5 feet, then add 5 pounds for each additional inch of height.

A more accurate measure of ideal and excessive weight is body mass index (BMI), a weight-to-height index. BMI can be determined by dividing your weight in kilograms by the square of your height in meters (kg/m²). A BMI index of 19 to 24 is considered desirable, 25 to 29 indicates overweight, and over 30 indicates obesity. Table 6 conveniently presents height and weight standards for men and women of small, medium, and large frames (the weight of clothes and shoes were included).

Table 5. What's Your Body Mass Index (BMI)?

Healthy		Overweight					Obese				
BMI 19	24	25	26	27	28	29	30	35	40	45	50
Height				Weight in pounds							
4' 10″ 91	115	119	124	129	134	138	143	167	191	215	239
4' 11″ 94	119	124	128	133	138	143	148	173	198	222	247
5' 0″ 97	123	128	133	138	143	148	153	179	204	230	255
5' 1″ 100	127	132	137	143	148	153	158	185	211	238	264
5' 2″ 104	131	136	142	147	153	158	164	191	218	246	273
5' 3″ 107	135	141	146	152	158	163	169	197	225	254	282
5' 4″ 110	140	145	151	157	163	169	174	204	232	262	291
5' 5″ 114	144	150	156	162	168	174	180	210	240	270	300
5' 6″ 118	148	155	161	167	173	179	186	216	247	278	309
5' 7″ 121	153	159	166	172	178	185	191	223	255	287	319
5' 8″ 125	158	164	171	177	184	190	197	230	262	295	328
5' 9″ 128	162	169	176	182	189	196	203	236	270	304	338
5' 10″ 132	167	174	181	188	195	202	209	243	278	313	348
5' 11″ 136	172	179	186	193	200	208	215	250	286	322	358
6' 0″ 140	177	184	191	199	206	213	221	258	294	331	368
6' 1″ 144	182	189	197	204	212	219	227	265	302	340	378
6' 2″ 148	186	194	202	210	218	225	233	272	311	350	389
6' 3″ 152	192	200	208	216	224	232	240	279	319	359	399
6' 4″ 156	197	205	213	221	230	238	246	287	328	369	410

(Source: Modified from National Institutes of Health. *Clinical Guidelines on the Identification, Evaluation, and Treatment of Overweight and Obesity in Adults.* Mayo Clinic on High Blood Pressure, 1998.)

Table 6. Height and Weight Standards

Men				Women			
Height	Small	Medium	Large	Height	Small	Medium	Large
5' 2"	128–134	131–141	138–150	4' 10"	102–111	109–121	118–131
5' 3"	130–136	133–143	140–153	4' 11"	103–113	111–123	120–134
5' 4"	132–138	135–145	142–156	5' 0"	104–115	113–126	122–137
5' 5"	134–140	137–148	144–160	5' 1"	106–118	115–129	125–140
5' 6"	136–142	139–151	146–164	5' 2"	108–121	118–132	128–143
5' 7"	138–145	142–154	149–168	5' 3"	111–124	121–135	131–147
5' 8"	140–148	145–157	152–172	5' 4"	114–127	124–138	134–151
5' 9"	142–151	148–160	155–176	5' 5"	117–130	127–141	137–155
5' 10"	144–154	151–163	158–180	5' 6"	120–133	130–144	140–159
5' 11"	146–157	154–166	161–184	5' 7"	123–136	133–147	143–163
6' 0"	149–160	157–170	164–188	5' 8"	126–139	136–150	146–167
6' 1"	152–164	160–174	168–192	5' 9"	129–142	139–153	149–170
6' 2"	155–168	164–178	172–197	5' 10"	132–145	142–156	152–173
6' 3"	158–172	167–182	176–202	5' 11"	135–148	145–159	155–176
6' 4"	162–176	171–187	181–207	6' 0"	138–151	148–162	158–179

Of particular interest is the fact that the body shape of obese people is a predictor of health risks. Fat that is confined mainly to the waist (which has been likened to an "apple-shape") occurs more commonly in men and portends a higher risk for atherosclerosis, heart disease, hypertension, stroke, and diabetes. Fat in this area is metabolically very active; that is, it is released into the circulation and may accumulate in your arteries. A waist circumference of more than 40 inches in men, or 35 inches in women, is considered a health risk. If fat is mainly confined to the hips, buttocks, and thighs, imparting a "pear-shaped" body, then it appears to confer no greater health risks than in people of normal weight. This configuration is seen more frequently in women. Fat in this location is metabolically inactive and does not cause arterial damage.

In fewer than 5 percent of cases, obesity can be traced to hormonal disorders. Several factors are known to influence weight gain:

- *Genes* play a role in energy metabolism. With a family history of obesity, children have a 25 to 30 percent greater chance of being obese. Also, the weight of adopted children seems to correlate with the weight of their true parents rather than that of their foster parents.

- *Gender* also plays a role in energy metabolism. For example, the greater muscle mass in men burns 10 to 20 percent more calories than in women at rest.

- *Aging* is accompanied by a decrease in muscle mass and a slowing of metabolism.

- *Overfeeding* in childhood may increase the number of fat cells and set the stage for lifelong obesity.

- *Quitting smoking* is accompanied by a reduced metabolic rate.

- *Physical inactivity* reduces energy expenditure, so that fewer calories are burned.

- *High-fat diets* increase weight by providing more calories than diets consisting mainly of protein and carbohydrate, with limited fat. Even when calories are the same, however, more fat is stored in fat tissue when the diet is high in fat.

Numerous endocrine and metabolic consequences of abdominal obesity (based on waist circumference) have been identified. They account for the predisposition to diabetes and atherosclerosis. In particular, the combination of abdominal obesity, diabetes, elevated blood glucose when fasting, or high levels of cholesterol and triglyceride fat in the blood and hypertension had been dubbed the "the deadly quartet," but the combination is now known as "Metabolic Syndrome." This combination of metabolic and endocrine disturbance is also marked by a decreased sensitivity to the metabolic action of insulin.

In the final analysis, obesity results from an excessive consumption of calories and/or an insufficient expenditure of energy. Although the latter condition may result from a lack of physical activity, energy expenditure also depends on body metabolism, which is genetically determined. You can't do anything about your genes, but you can control your weight by monitoring your eating habits and physical activity. It is up to you to take charge of and protect your health by maintaining a normal weight.

48 What Is the Best Way to Lose Excess Weight, and Are Diet Pills Indicated?

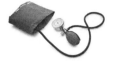

Persuading overweight and obese patients to reduce their weight is one of the most frustrating and difficult problems that doctors face. Although doctors particularly recognize how important weight control is for the health of their patients (see Question 47), far too often patients seem unable to make a sustained commitment to reduce their weight, despite knowledge of the health risks. The single most important factor for a successful weight-loss program is the patient's motivation. Effective treatment of excess weight or obesity is also fraught with frustration and emotional tension for patients. Americans spend more than $30 billion each year trying to stay trim and thin, and in an effort to lose excess weight. As a nation we obviously find it difficult to do these things.

Altering lifestyle and eating patterns requires both mental and physical energy (see Questions 40, 46, 47). The combination of decreased caloric intake and increased caloric expenditure through increased physical activity with aerobic exercise (requiring active physical motion and increased oxygen consumption) are the keys to successful weight loss. Reducing the number of fatty meals and dairy products consumed are basic. Ideally, one should limit fat to no more than 30 percent of the total calories in the diet.

Adequate exercise can prove very significant in preventing excess weight from recurring. Moderate or mild exercise — walking, golfing, jogging, bicycling, playing tennis, cross-country skiing, swimming, engaging in calisthenics, dancing, or taking exercise classes — may be sufficient to keep the weight off if the activity is performed several times weekly. For example, some people will find that a brisk walk for thirty minutes most days of the week is very helpful. But many individuals are most motivated to exercise when they take part in group activities. Regardless of the type of exercise you choose, your workout should be enjoyable; otherwise, you won't stay with it.

> The combination of decreased caloric intake and increased caloric expenditure through increased physical activity with aerobic exercise (requiring active physical motion and increased oxygen consumption) are the keys to successful weight loss.

Modest exercise can reduce weight and lower blood pressure just as effectively as strenuous exercise. But before embarking on any strenuous exercise program, it is prudent to talk to your doctor. To date, no evidence shows that vigorous exercise is more beneficial than regularly performed, moderate exercise. Aerobic exercise should be started slowly, with the duration and intensity being gradually increased. There is little reason to perform strenuous isometric exercises such as heavy weight lifting, which is used to strengthen muscles and "body-build." Very strenuous exercise can raise blood pressure to dangerously high levels, especially in people with hypertension.

It is noteworthy that men typically eat more than women, because the greater muscle mass in men uses more energy. Under normal circumstances, men burn 10 to 20 percent more calories than do women. But, as both genders will discover, aging and the expected decrease in muscle mass are accompanied by a decrease in metabolism, which in turn is followed by weight gain.

Set a realistic time frame and goal for weight reduction. A desirable goal is one that will reduce blood pressure, cholesterol, and blood sugar, assuming they are elevated. Gradual loss of weight (for example, 1 pound per week) is recommended, because this goal is attainable and such a pattern is most likely to succeed in permanent weight reduction. To determine how many calories you can eat daily and still lose one pound each week, try the following: Multiply your weight in pounds by 10. For example, if you weigh 160 pounds, 160 multiplied by 10 equals 1,600 calories. You should consume no more than this daily in order to lose one pound per week.

Here is how to do it: Change your eating habits, eat less, and avoid excess calories and fat, which are often consumed in the form of "fast foods." A diet focused on lean meat, fish, chicken, and turkey without the skin, along with more grains, fruits, and vegetables can

> Consumption of lean meat, fish, chicken, and turkey without the skin, and more grains, fruits, and vegetables can provide an excellent balance.

provide an excellent balance. Recently, the *Dietary Approaches to Stop Hypertension* (DASH) study demonstrated that a diet stressing fruits, vegetables, grains, and low-fat items (accounting for less than 30 percent of total calories) significantly reduced blood pressure in hypertensive patients and those with borderline elevations (see Question 49); it also promoted weight loss. The diet was rich in potassium, calcium, magnesium, and fiber.

A modest increase in the consumption of water or nonfattening beverages, along with the consumption of high-fiber foods may help curb the appetite. Snacking between meals must be avoided; it may help to eat carrot and celery sticks if the urge to snack is particularly strong. Alcohol consumption in men should be limited to no more than 2 ounces of whiskey, 10 ounces of wine (two wine glasses), or 24 ounces of beer (two cans) daily; women and thin people should consume even less alcohol. Alcohol is a source of nonnutritional calories, which can increase weight; furthermore, exceeding the recommended limits can increase blood pressure. It has been reported that excessive alcohol consumption may account for the elevated blood pressure in 7 to 10 percent of the hypertensive population.

A number of "crash" or novelty diets are designed to help people lose weight rapidly, and some of these diets work. However, some may prove to be hazardous and ineffective for long-term weight loss. Really, who can consume all their meals from liquid drinks or specially prepared packaged foods or exclude whole classes of foods from their diets? Eating should be an enjoyable experience, not an obsession. The key is moderation in all food choices; consume only the calories needed to sustain ideal weight. This is balanced with moderate exercise, which burns calories.

A healthy diet consists of a variety of foods. It yields approximately 30 percent or less fat, about 60 percent carbohydrate with very little refined sugar, and about 10 percent protein.

The late Dr. Robert Atkins advocated the use of diets high in protein and fat and low in carbohydrates (that is, no more than 20 percent of total calories) for weight reduction. Although this diet can curb the appetite, reduce caloric intake, cause weight loss, and even lower blood cholesterol in some people, many other people find it difficult to adhere to a low-carbohydrate diet. Such a diet bans fruit and fruit juice, bread, grains, potato, rice, corn, dairy products (other than cheese, cream, or butter), and sugar in any form. If carbohydrates are not strictly limited, dieters following this plan may fail to lose weight and experience significantly increased cholesterol levels. It is noteworthy that most Asians are not obese, yet they consume diets high in carbohydrates.

Dr. Dean Ornish advocates an almost fat-free diet — similar to a strict vegetarian diet — for weight loss. Many individuals cannot adhere to this diet, and vitamin and iron deficiency may occur without proper supplementation of these substances.

Over-the-counter appetite suppressants should be used with caution. They can stimulate the nervous system and may increase blood pressure; in addition, they do not suppress appetites for long periods of time. One setback in the search for an effective appetite suppressant occurred in 1997 when it was reported that the appetite suppressant "fen-phen" — the combination of fenfluramine (Pondimin) or dexfenfluramine (Redux) and phentermine — caused thickening and sometimes malfunctioning of heart valves in an alarming number of patients consuming this drug for weight reduction. Six million Americans had used fen-phen.

Orlistat (Xenical), which prevents absorption of 30 percent of dietary fat, has been approved by the U.S. Food and Drug Administration for long-term treatment of obesity. This drug should be considered as an aid for some obese patients who are resistant to weight-loss programs, especially individuals with hypertension, diabetes, and/or elevated levels of fats in their blood. It is recommended that orlistat be taken three times daily with each meal containing fat; it can be omitted if the meal does not include fat.

Orlistat appears modestly effective in promoting weight loss and should be considered for use with some very obese patients; however, it frequently causes bloating, flatulence, oily stools, diarrhea and fecal urgency, and incontinence. Furthermore, it interferes with the absorption of the fat-soluble vitamins A, D, E, and K and beta-carotene; replacement of fat-soluble vitamins, with the supplements being consumed two hours before or after orlistat, is indicated in patients taking orlistat. The side effects associated with this drug may be minimized by reducing fat in the diet.

Surgical procedures to reduce the amount of food absorbed from the intestines are a last resort for obese individuals who are unable to lose weight in another way. However, this procedure, although effective for weight loss, has numerous possible side effects. It should be used only when all else has failed and obesity is extreme — that is, if the BMI is 35 or more.

Weight reduction can do wonders for your physical and mental health, and it may also improve your energy level. Motivation and commitment to a weight-loss program, of course, are essential ingredients for success. It is up to you!

49 What Is the Best Diet for Treating Hypertension and Its Complications? What Are the "Mediterranean" and "DASH" Diets?

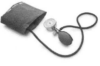

The best diet for people with hypertension satisfies the following criteria:

- It allows the person to avoid becoming overweight or obese, and it maintains weight near the normal acceptable standard range.
- It limits total sodium intake to 2,400 mg of sodium per day.
- It limits alcohol consumption to no more than two drinks of wine, beer, or spirits per day.
- It helps lower "bad" cholesterol (LDL or low-density lipoprotein) and fat levels (triglycerides), if they are elevated.
- It includes food with minerals (especially potassium) that tend to lower blood pressure (BP).

The importance of losing excess body weight for hypertensive patients and the best means of losing weight are discussed in detail elsewhere in this book (see Questions 47 and 48). Here we emphasize, once again, that weight loss is best achieved by reducing caloric consumption (with less than 30 percent fat in the diet) and by increasing caloric expenditure through regular, moderate exercise performed for thirty minutes most days per week. Reducing the total number of calories in the diet is essential and can be achieved by reducing fat consumption; 1 gram of fat is equivalent to 9 calories, whereas 1 gram of protein or carbohydrate is equivalent to only 4 calories. Weight loss of even a few pounds may reduce BP. Indeed, weight loss is certainly one of the most effective ways of reducing BP without drugs.

Restricting total sodium consumption to no more than 2,400 mg per day can also reduce BP in hypertensive individuals who are salt sensitive — that is, those who develop hypertension when they consume excess amounts of salt (see Question 34). This may account for 50 to 60 percent of the hypertensive population. Most African Americans are especially sensitive to salt. Approximately 75 percent of sodium consumed comes from processed food (that is, food prepared by a food company for public consumption). Only a relatively small percentage is found in unprocessed food (that is, naturally occurring food to which nothing has been added), and only 15 percent is usually added to home cooking or at the table. It is especially important to read food labels and become aware of foods that have a high concentration of sodium (above 400 mg in each serving) so that you can avoid them. Even some local water supplies may have a high content of sodium.

There are numerous acceptable salt substitutes (which contain less sodium than normal salt). Any salt substitute containing potassium should be used with caution in individuals with impaired kidney function, as retention of excessive amounts of potassium can damage the electrical impulses and function of the heart. Potassium-containing salt substitutes should not be used without careful monitoring by a doctor in individuals receiving a potassium-sparing diuretic or other drugs (ACE inhibitors, ARBs, direct renin inhibitors) that may cause retention of potassium, as their consumption could elevate potassium in the blood to harmful levels. Fruits and vegetables are an excellent source of potassium, but intake of these foods should be watched in patients on these drugs and in those with impaired kidney function to avoid a dangerous increase of potassium in the blood.

> *Potassium-containing salt substitutes should be used with caution in individuals with impaired kidney function and should not be used at all in individuals receiving a potassium-sparing diuretic.*

Excessive alcohol consumption is responsible for hypertension in 7 to 10 percent of all cases (see Question 24). This hypertension appears to result from stimulation of the brain and nervous system, which in turn causes constriction of the arterioles. Women with hypertension should consume less alcohol than hypertensive men, because women are usually smaller and metabolize alcohol less efficiently than men do. It should be appreciated that alcohol adds calories to the diet, which is undesirable for a person who is trying to lose weight. Evidence suggests, however, that limited alcohol consumption protects individuals from heart attacks and artery damage when compared to those who do not drink alcohol. The beneficial effects conferred by consumption of modest amounts of alcohol seem to result from improvements in cholesterol concentrations; alcohol may slightly increase HDL, or "good" cholesterol, levels.

Elevated LDL, or "bad" cholesterol, levels and probably elevated triglyceride (another lipid) levels in the blood increase the risk of heart attacks, stroke, and hardening of the arteries. In the presence of hypertension, the risk of these complications is significantly increased, which makes it all the more important to reduce the level of these fats in addition to normalizing BP.

A reduction of LDLs and triglycerides may be accomplished in several ways:

- Reduce consumption of dietary cholesterol and fats (by limiting consumption of fat to no more that 30 percent of caloric intake).
- Lose weight, if overweight.
- Take cholesterol- and fat-lowering drugs, if indicated.

Some foods contain cholesterol and harmful fats, especially saturated fats (found in animal fats, lard, dairy products, chocolate, coconut and palm oil, and some vegetable shortening), and trans-fatty acids (found in margarine and in crackers, cookies, and cakes). These fats should be avoided but can be replaced when necessary with monounsaturated fats, particularly olive oil. It is noteworthy that people in Spain, France, Italy, and Greece, whose diets tend to include lots of olive oil, vegetables, fruits, and grains but little saturated fat and processed foods (a diet known as the "Mediterranean diet") have relatively little heart disease. Polyunsaturated fats, such as corn, sunflower, safflower, and soybean oil, are also far healthier than saturated fats. Nevertheless, all oils are fats and can add a significant amount of calories if used too frequently or in too-high quantities. If weight loss and diet are unable to sufficiently lower LDL cholesterol and triglyceride levels, then drug treatment may be indicated.

The Dietary Approaches to Stop Hypertension (DASH) diet has been found to be effective in lowering BP in hypertensive individuals (see Questions 48 and 97). The DASH diet consists of 27 percent calories from fat, lots of fruits and vegetables (eight to ten servings daily), low-fat or nonfat dairy products, nuts, grains, fiber, and small amounts of meat, fish, and poultry. After eight weeks on the DASH diet, the systolic and diastolic pressures in hypertensive individuals participating in this study decreased by 11.4 and 5.5 mm Hg, respectively. Even people with high-normal BPs experienced a decrease of about 3.5 mm Hg in their systolic and 2 mm Hg in their diastolic pressure. The significant decrease in BP found with the DASH diet occurred without any other lifestyle changes, indicating the value of decreasing fat and increasing consumption of minerals, which are abundant in fruits and vegetables.

> The DASH diet has been found to be effective in lowering blood pressure in hypertensive individuals and has been recommended as a very healthy diet for all Americans.

Experimental and clinical studies suggest that increased consumption of potassium is valuable in gradually reducing BP and preventing stroke. The potassium content of the DASH diet is roughly 2½ times that consumed in an ordinary diet in the United States. There is also evidence that vegetables may play a role in reducing BP by releasing a chemical (nitric oxide) into the blood that dilates blood vessels. People with impaired kidney function should talk to their doctor about consuming large quantities of foods high in potassium or potassium-substituted salts, since retaining excess amounts of potassium can impair the function of the heart and cause an irregular heartbeat and even death.

The roles played by other minerals found in fruits and vegetables (such as calcium and magnesium) and by fat reduction in decreasing BP are less clear. Potentially, the DASH diet could actually prevent hypertension in some individuals. At any rate, the DASH diet is an extremely healthy diet that should be recommended to all Americans. For individuals with high BP, we recommend limiting sodium to 1,500 mg daily (although this is good guideline for everyone to follow).

50 Is Garlic or Fish Oil Good for You if Your Blood Pressure or Cholesterol Is Elevated?

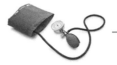

Any food purported to benefit people with hypertension or high levels of blood cholesterol should have its claims validated by scientific evaluation before the medical profession advises its use or the public accepts it. The claims of the beneficial effects from many "health foods" are unsubstantiated and often fraudulent, and consuming them may result in an enormous financial investment without any reward.

Although the beneficial effects of garlic on blood pressure and cholesterol were controversial and inconclusive for many years, more recently several studies involving about 1,000 people reported that taking 600 to 1,000 mg daily of garlic supplements lowered total cholesterol by 9 to 12 percent. Consumption of garlic also caused levels of triglycerides (another fat in the blood, which may be harmful) to decrease, but high-density lipoprotein (HDL, or "good," cholesterol) remained unchanged. Furthermore, it has been reported that even 500 mg of garlic supplement taken daily for seven years protected arteries from becoming stiff and hardened by deposits of cholesterol when compared to the arteries of people not taking the garlic. Allicin, an oil in gar-

Garlic supplements appear to lower total cholesterol and triglycerides, but they do not affect "good" (HDL) cholesterol levels.

lic, was reported to be responsible for lowering cholesterol in the blood. However, other investigators could not confirm this.

Several studies have reported that garlic — usually in the form of deodorized powder — lowers blood pressure. However, a recent extensive review of studies on the therapeutic values of garlic indicates that garlic does not have any antihypertensive action. Other ways of lowering cholesterol and blood pressure are much more effective, reliable, and practical.

A few years ago, reports claimed that fish oil was good for lowering cholesterol and blood pressure and would protect against heart attack. Eskimos, who eat large amounts of fish, whale, and seal meat (all of which contain high quantities of fish oil), have relatively low total cholesterol and triglycerides in their blood and a decreased tendency for their blood to clot. In addition, Eskimos have significantly fewer heart attacks than non-Eskimos who do not consume a diet high in fish oil. As a result of enthusiastic reports regarding the beneficial effects of fish oil, the sale of fish-oil capsules soared.

Fish oil contains omega-3 polyunsaturated fatty acids, which occur naturally in fish and are especially abundant in tuna, mackerel, trout, and salmon. Such fatty acids are important in forming chemicals in humans that can lower cholesterol and triglycerides and can increase HDL.

Fish oil capsules are available in several commercial preparations. Large doses, however, are required to produce a beneficial effect on blood pressure and blood triglycerides; little or no change occurs in the LDL, or "bad," cholesterol. Unfortunately, very large doses have been linked to a risk of bleeding, and the high concentrations of vitamin A and D contained in fish oil can be toxic. Capsules of fish oil are, of course, high in fat and calories — characteristics that are undesirable if you are trying to lose weight — and they may cause intestinal upset and have an unpleasant fishy aftertaste. Fortunately, eating fish several times per week may be just as effective in lowering blood pressure and reducing levels of cholesterol and fats in the blood as consuming capsules of fish oil. In one study, eating two cans of mackerel daily for two weeks decreased systolic and diastolic blood pressure by 15 and 7 mm Hg, respectively; decreased total cholesterol by 7 percent and triglycerides by 50 percent; and increased HDL, or "good," cholesterol.

The American Heart Association and experts managing hypertension and cholesterol and fat abnormalities in the blood have concluded that eating fish several times each week may reduce the risk of vascular disease and possibly protect against heart attack and stroke. Because large doses of omega-3 fatty acids are required for any beneficial therapeutic effect, and because toxic side effects are possible, prolonged use of supplements is not recommended. Frequent consumption of fish, however, is highly desirable.

51 Must I Give Up Smoking Because of My Hypertension?

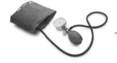

The answer to this question is an emphatic "yes"! There is no more treacherous contributor to health problems than cigarette smoking. Even smoke from cigar or pipes is hazardous to your health. The havoc caused by smoking is monumental, and it is the most preventable cause of premature death in the United States. It causes more than 1,100 deaths per day and 20 percent of all deaths, and smoking-related medical care costs approximately $50 billion annually. In addition, 15 percent of people who smoke cigarettes develop lung cancer.

Smoking accounts for several alarming statistics:

- 30 percent of cardiovascular deaths (including heart attack, heart failure, stroke, and blood vessel damage)
- 30 percent of all cancer deaths (including 87 percent of lung cancer deaths)
- 80 percent of deaths from chronic obstructive lung disease (primarily emphysema)

Consider this sobering fact: Smoking cigarettes causes lung and laryngeal cancer, chronic bronchitis, coronary heart disease, hardening of the arteries (atherosclerosis), cancer of the mouth and esophagus, chronic obstructive lung disease, low-birth-weight babies, unsuccessful pregnancies, increased infant mortality, and peptic ulcer. It may be a contributing factor for the development of cancer of the urinary bladder, pancreas, kidneys, and stomach. It addition, smoking appears to be associated with stroke and possibly cataracts, bowel disease, macular degeneration, and breast cancer. And it can decrease the "good" cholesterol (HDL) and increase the "bad" cholesterol (LDL) in your blood. It may also cause a tendency for platelets (small blood cells) to aggregate and form clots that could block the circulation and cause a heart attack or stroke.

Smoking a pipe or cigars may be less injurious to a person's health than inhaling cigarette smoke. Nevertheless, these forms of smoking still pose a significant risk not only to the smoker but to all those who inhale the smoke passively.

The nicotine in cigarettes increases your heart rate and constricts your blood vessels, which may raise your blood pressure for ten minutes to one hour. Roughly one-third of all hypertensives smoke. Nicotine is believed to lessen the effectiveness of some antihypertensive drugs, particularly the beta blockers. Although smoking does not cause permanent hypertension, the repeated temporary elevations of blood pressure associated with it may prove harmful.

The late Dr. Thomas Pickering, using ambulatory blood pressure monitoring for twenty-four hours, demonstrated that, during the day, systolic pressures were 5 to 10 mm Hg higher in one-pack-a-day smokers than in nonsmokers; at night there was no difference in pressures between smokers and nonsmokers. Based on his findings, smoking even one pack per day appears to be responsible for a mildly elevated blood pressure in normal healthy subjects — clearly demonstrating the negative effect of nicotine.

It seems reasonable to suggest that this daytime smoking-related increase would augment the blood pressure of hypertensive individuals and increase the risk of serious complications.

Nicotine activates the sympathetic nervous system and releases hormones (epinephrine and norepinephrine) into the circulation that not only increase your heart rate and blood pressure but may also cause irregular heartbeats. In addition, smoking decreases the supply of oxygen to tissues and vital organs. It adds carbon monoxide to the blood, which may damage blood vessels, permit cholesterol accumulation in the arteries, and accelerate atherosclerosis. Indeed, the arteries of the heart (coronary arteries) are more frequently and more severely damaged in smokers than they are in nonsmokers.

Although heavy or chain-smokers are at greater risk than light smokers for developing the diseases mentioned above, nonsmokers who are exposed to cigarette smoke from others (from "second-hand smoking") are also at increased risk for heart and lung disease. People living with a smoker have a 30 percent greater chance of developing heart disease than if they were not exposed to smoke. Such second-hand smoking is estimated to cause 37,000 deaths yearly. Children of parents who smoke are more likely to suffer from lung infections and asthma than children who are not exposed to smoke.

Cigarette smokers without any health problems are two to three times more likely to have a heart attack than nonsmokers, and the odds of surviving a heart attack are usually worse in those who smoke. The presence of high blood pressure, elevated blood cholesterol, diabetes, or obesity all further increase the risk of heart attack, stroke, and blood vessel damage (hardening of the arteries with a blockage and/or rupture of these vessels). Smokers with hypertension are three to five times more likely to die from a heart attack or heart failure than nonsmokers and twice as likely to die of a stroke. As the number of risk factors increases, so too does the risk of premature death; with each additional risk factor, the chance of death may double. If all risk factors are present, the chance of premature death is enormous.

The good news is that 40 million Americans have given up smoking, and it is extremely rare to see a physician who smokes. Unfortunately, another 30 million Americans continue to smoke. Sadly the number of teenagers who smoke is increasing — especially young women. Psychosocial (that is, emotional and social) experiences and peer pressure play a central role in influencing the attitudes of many teenagers. Some young women apparently use cigarettes to stay slim, as smoking increases body metabolism and can curb the appetite (see Question 52).

Additional good news is that one year after quitting smoking, the risk of cardiovascular disease diminishes markedly; at the same time, the risk of heart disease decreases by about 50 percent, and five years after quitting the risk is almost the same as in non-smokers. The risk of lung and other cancers, strokes, and chronic lung diseases decreases as well but never returns to the level of those who never smoked. After ten to fifteen years of abstinence, the risk of death from a smoking-related disease is nearly as low as that of people who never smoked.

Quitting cigarette smoking is the most effective and important life insurance policy available. For your own sake and for the health of your family and all those with whom you come in contact, give it up!

52 What Is the Best Way to Quit Smoking?

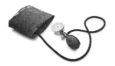

With any form of addiction, whether it be addiction to alcohol, drugs, or cigarette smoking, *motivation* is absolutely essential in quitting. Without sufficient commitment, the smoking cessation plan has little, if any, chance of success. To underscore the importance of motivation, note that 95 percent of the 40 million people who have quit smoking have done it on their own. The poor success rates of many formal smoking cessation programs are most likely related to insufficient motivation (see Question 51).

It is usually not easy to quit smoking, especially for the heavy smoker, because most smokers are both physically and psychologically addicted. However, the fear of disease caused by cigarette smoking, plus increases in tobacco taxes, have had a significant effect on Americans, and tobacco consumption has decreased by 50 percent during the past thirty years. Ironically, the macho male model who appeared in Marlboro cigarette ads many years ago died of lung cancer. Unfortunately, the seriousness of the health hazards of smoking has not been sufficiently transmitted to populations outside of the United States, where smoking remains prevalent at all levels of society and in all professions.

> With any form of addiction, whether it be addiction to alcohol, drugs, or cigarette smoking, motivation is absolutely essential in quitting.

Millions of Americans try to give up smoking each year, but only 10 percent are successful on the first attempt. Persistence plus firm motivation are the keys to success. Nearly two-thirds of all people who repeatedly try to quit eventually succeed. Also, it is never too late to quit, given that health benefits may be gained by abstaining from this habit, no matter what the age of the individual and no matter how long they have been smoking cigarettes.

There is no magic formula for smoking cessation. Some smokers will respond to one approach better than another. Although smoking is physically addictive due to the activity of nicotine and other products introduced into cigarettes, it also results in strong psychological and social dependence because it becomes associated with a large variety of situations and emotional states. Stressful situations may be lessened and concentration improved by smoking, which makes it especially desirable under some circumstances. Repeatedly smoking at a particular time of the day, under a variety of emotionally stressful circumstances, and during special social events and periods of entertainment can cause the habit to become ingrained and trigger the desire to automatically smoke at these times.

For smoking cessation to be most successful, certain steps should be followed. Deviation from these guidelines may be desired by some smokers, however, and may not doom the effort to quit.

First, an earnest desire to quit smoking is essential. One should be prepared to experience short-term discomfort (irritability, anxiety, and loss of concentration), which becomes most noticeable 2 to 4 days after cessation but usually disappears within 10 to 14 days. Thereafter, the desire to smoke may periodically occur months or years later, but this urge to smoke usually lasts only a few seconds. It is extremely important to appreciate that anyone who has been a heavy smoker cannot become a "social smoker." Any "slip" — even smoking one cigarette — is very likely to cause full resumption of smoking (much like what can happen to former chronic alcoholics or former cocaine or heroine addicts). Relapses are most likely to occur during negative emotional states, particularly within the first few months after quitting.

In general, the following suggestions and approaches to smoking cessation have proved helpful:

1. *Consider the importance of quitting and list the health hazards of smoking and the important reasons you wish to quit.* Enlist the help of others — especially your family and friends — to give moral support and ask them to avoid smoking in your presence. Make a list of locations and situations when you are most likely to smoke and be prepared to either avoid these circumstances or cope with them. Each day, check the reasons you want to quit. Then designate a date on which to quit, preferably a day when your stress level is low and you face few problems and pressures.

2. *Stopping abruptly seems more effective than trying to cut down gradually.* Throw away all cigarettes and matches. The use of Zyban (bupropion, Wellbutrin), an antidepressant, has proved

valuable in some smokers because this drug reduces the desire to smoke, even in people who are not depressed. Another drug, Chantix (varenicline), may also help, acting to block the effect of nicotine; however, it may sometimes worsen or cause a psychiatric illness. These drugs require a prescription, and the dosage and schedule for use should be left to your physician.

Nicotine replacement may be especially helpful in heavy smokers who are addicted. Nicotine transdermal patches (such as Habitrol, Nicoderm, and Prostep) offer significant advantages over nicotine chewing gum (Nicorette): The former products are easier to use, cause fewer side effects, and deliver a more constant and adequate dose of nicotine. Although nicotine patches can be purchased without a prescription, you should consult with your physician regarding dosage schedules, especially when patches are used in combination with Zyban. Other forms of nicotine delivery — by means of a nasal spray or inhaler, for example — appear to be much less effective than patches and chewing gums containing nicotine.

You must not smoke if you are using a nicotine replacement, because smoking might significantly elevate the nicotine concentration in the blood and cause problems, especially in individuals with heart disease. Anecdotal reports suggesting that nicotine patches may cause heart irregularities and even heart attacks or strokes have caused concern; a study of male volunteers, however, revealed no differences in side effects between subjects using nicotine patches and those using patches without nicotine.

The value of hypnosis and acupuncture is poorly substantiated as a means of smoking cessation, although some people have benefited from these treatments.

The Ongoing Urge to Smoke

Be prepared to cope with the urge to smoke, which is especially strong at the beginning of withdrawal. Changing routine activities may be very helpful. Avoid locations and situations where you routinely smoke. Perform activities to divert your attention such as exercising, taking a walk immediately after meals, going to a movie, joining friends who are strongly opposed to smoking, chewing ordinary gum, sucking on mints, or eating celery, carrot sticks, or unsalted pretzels. You should avoid substituting high-calorie foods for cigarettes, because smoking cessation decreases the body's metabolism and leads to a tendency to gain weight. Continually recall the health hazards of smoking, including death from heart disease, lung disease, stroke, or a variety of cancers. For female smokers, this list also includes risks to the fetus during pregnancy.

Some smokers may be helped by formal cessation programs with group interaction and mutual support. You must always remember that the key to quitting depends almost entirely on the strength of your desire to quit. If you fail to quit on the first attempt, always try again. *Remember, no one ever died from trying to quit smoking.*

53 Are Atherosclerosis and Arteriosclerosis the Same? What Do They Result in and Can They Cause Hypertension?

Atherosclerosis affects the larger arteries, and arteriosclerosis affects the smaller ones. For practical purposes they are the same — and both are treacherous. These conditions may lead to blockage of the arteries (heart attacks and strokes), kidney disease, amputations (especially of the lower extremities), and aneurysms (weakened areas in the arterial wall that expand like a balloon and sometimes rupture). Both atherosclerosis and arteriosclerosis are aggravated by high blood pressure, high blood

> *For practical purposes, atherosclerosis and arteriosclerosis are the same—and both are treacherous. These conditions may lead to blockage of the arteries, kidney disease, amputations, and aneurysms.*

cholesterol, and cigarette smoking. They are particularly common in countries where consumption of dairy and animal products is high and where hypertension is common. Reducing blood pressure, lowering cholesterol, and stopping smoking will slow down the sclerotic process. People who do not have diabetes, high blood pressure, or high cholesterol, and who do not smoke cigarettes, usually have less atherosclerosis or arteriosclerosis.

With the modern diets typical of industrialized societies, hardening of the arteries occurs with aging and results in increased systolic pressure (see Questions 22 and 37). Over time the large arteries become hardened and lose much of their elasticity, causing increased resistance to the blood expelled by the heart during contraction (systole). The hardening of the arteries that supply the kidneys can sometimes significantly impair blood flow to the kidneys, which may then release renin, an enzyme that is converted to angiotensin, a hormone that causes constriction of arterioles and thereby leads to hypertension (see Question 38).

54 Should High Blood Pressure Be Treated Differently in Men Versus Women, and in African Americans Versus White People?

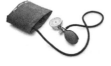

Prior to beginning menopause, women are less likely than men of comparable age to be hypertensive, and their risk of heart attack and stroke is less than that in men of comparable age. After menopause, however, the protective effect of estrogen is lost. Consequently, the frequency of high blood pressure is as great, if not greater, in postmenopausal women than in men of comparable age. Furthermore, older women have as many heart attacks and strokes as do elderly men. For these reasons, it is important to treat high blood pressure in men and women of any age and to seek out and treat other risk factors for cardiovascular disease such as cigarette smoking, diabetes mellitus, and high cholesterol.

No convincing evidence exists to suggest that any of the drugs that lower blood pressure are more effective in one gender than in the other.

It is well established that in any decade of life hypertension is more prevalent and more severe in African Americans — both men and women — than in whites. This leads to negative complications at an earlier age in African Americans (see Question 26). Young African-American men are particularly vulnerable to developing the devastating consequences of high blood pressure. And because men, whether African American or white, do not consult a doctor as frequently as women do, hypertension in African-American men may go undiscovered and untreated more often than in the white population.

> *None of these drugs that lower blood pressure appears to be more effective in one gender than in the other.*

For both men and women, diuretics and calcium-blocking drugs seem to be more effective in African Americans and older subjects than are the other drugs. However, this does not rule out the use of ACE inhibitors, angiotensin receptor blockers, direct renin inhibitors, and beta blockers in African Americans who have been shown to respond well to these drugs. Regardless, in most patients of either gender or race, multiple drugs will be necessary to control hypertension, especially when it is severe.

55 Once I Start Taking Medicine for High Blood Pressure, Do I Have to Take It Forever?

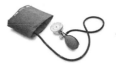

Usually you have to take antihypertensive drugs on a continuing basis if you want your blood pressure (BP) to remain normal. Medication to lower BP controls but does not cure hypertension. In this sense, hypertension is analogous to diabetes. Patients with diabetes must take pills or insulin to maintain their blood sugar in a normal range, but the therapy does not cure the diabetes.

Similarly, medication controls hypertension only so long as you take the drug.

Occasionally, well-motivated patients who keep their BPs well controlled with medication for more than two years will be able to gradually reduce the dose taken without any rise in BP. Some may wean themselves off of drugs altogether. This is particularly true for patients who modify their lifestyles so as to lose excess weight and then remain lean, exercise regularly, and consume very little salt. Most of the time, however, when patients stop taking their antihypertensive medications, their BP returns to the original, higher level. It may take days, weeks, or months for this to occur, depending upon how long BP has been adequately controlled. With prolonged use of a drug to control BP, the return of pressure to the formerly elevated level may take longer than if the medication were used for only a short period and then discontinued. If side effects are a reason for discontinuing the medication, you should consult your doctor — a different medication may be just as effective and offer fewer adverse effects.

56 Can Caffeine Be Harmful, and Should I Give It up if I Have Hypertension?

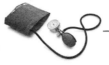

The consumption of coffee and tea is almost a ritual in practically all cultures and countries throughout the world. This ingrained behavior often adds to the zest of life, offering an opportunity for repeated social communication among friends and fellow workers. Many find it difficult and unpleasant to start the morning without coffee. Although the exhilaration of caffeine can account for some of this physical caffeine dependence, coffee drinking also provides psychological support to many. Coffee is a very important part of most adult lives, and it has been estimated that one-half of the population of the United States drinks three or more cups of coffee each day. Children do not, of course, share this need for morning coffee, but they may consume excess amounts of caffeine in soft drinks and chocolate to the point of causing nervousness, irritability, and an inability to relax.

Table 7 lists the concentration of caffeine in coffee, tea, soft drinks, chocolate, and "decaffeinated" drinks. In most people, caffeine increases alertness, concentration, and job performance, and it can lift one's mood. This effect may be accompanied by a *temporary* increase in heart rate and blood pressure in both hypertensive and normotensive people. One cup of strong coffee may increase diastolic blood pressure by 8 mm Hg in men with

Table 7. The Amounts of Caffeine in Some Common Foods and Beverages

Source		Caffeine (mg)
Coffee, ¾ cup (6 oz/180 mL)	Brewed, drip	103
	Instant	57
	Decaffeinated, brewed, and instant	2
Espresso (single)	Regular	100
	Decaffeinated	5
Tea, ¾ cup (6 oz/180 mL)	Black, brewed 3 minutes	40
	Instant	30
	Decaffeinated	1
Soft drinks, 1½ cups (12 oz/360 mL)	Cola type, regular and diet	31–70
	Noncola type	0–55
Chocolate	Cocoa, dry powder, 1 tablespoon	10
	Baking chocolate, 1 ounce (30 g)	25
	Chocolate milk, 1 cup (8 oz/250 mL)	10
	Milk chocolate bar, 1½ ounces (45 g)	10

(Source: Jean A.T. Pennington, Anna De Planter Bowes, and Helen Nichols Church. *Bowes and Church's Food Values of Portions Commonly Used*.17th ed. [Lippincott-Raven Publishers, 1998]. By permission.)

mild hypertension, whereas an increase of 3 mm Hg may occur in individuals with normal blood pressure. Furthermore, excess caffeine consumption can cause nervousness, irritability, anxiety, shakiness, panic attacks, insomnia, and an inability to relax and concentrate. If you want to decrease excessive caffeine consumption, proceed gradually so as to prevent headaches and other side effects that may result from reducing caffeine intake suddenly.

> Excess caffeine consumption can cause nervousness, irritability, anxiety, shakiness, panic attacks, insomnia, and an inability to relax and concentrate. It may also produce a temporary increase in heart rate and blood pressure in both hypertensive and normotensive people.

To date, no evidence has been found to prove that constriction of blood vessels due to caffeine consumption damages arteries or leads to heart attacks or strokes. Because caffeine stimulates the heart muscle and accelerates the heart rate, however, it can produce extra heartbeats (extra systoles) and cause palpitations (an annoying sensation of a pronounced or irregular heartbeat). Furthermore, in individuals who have periodic irregular heartbeats (atrial fibrillation), this stimulant may increase the frequency of these episodes. Caffeine may also provoke heartburn, diarrhea, or constipation; aggravate ulcers in the stomach; and increase urination.

In the past few decades, consumption of decaffeinated coffee has increased dramatically, particularly with the advent of decaffeinated beans, which permit brewing and improve flavor to the point where most people cannot tell the difference between regular and decaffeinated coffee. Perhaps one in five coffee drinkers uses the decaffeinated form to avoid any effects of caffeine. In the Unites States, decaffeinated coffee is routinely made available wherever regular coffee is served. Indeed, only decaffeinated coffee is served following dinner at many social gatherings and private parties. The demand for decaffeinated tea and cola drinks has also increased somewhat. Obviously, if one has several cups of coffee and also drinks tea and caffeinated soft drinks during the day, the amount of caffeine consumed can be considerable and result in undesirable side effects. Thus, it is wise to keep track of your caffeinated drink consumption.

Although no strong evidence implicates caffeine as a cause of permanent hypertension, it is reasonable for people who already have hypertension to avoid repeated elevations of blood pressure, particularly if these are exacerbated by the consumption of caffeinated drinks. For people with hypertension who regularly consume considerable amounts of caffeine, it would be wise to check the effect of drinking a cup of regular coffee on their blood pressure and heart rate. If the elevations of blood pressure are pronounced (systolic or diastolic elevations of 5 to 10 mm Hg) or if the heart rate is markedly increased or irregularities occur, then it is recommended that the consumption of caffeinated drinks be significantly reduced or replaced with the consumption of decaffeinated drinks.

Many experts recommend that daily caffeine consumption be limited to about 200 mg per day (two cups of coffee, four cups of tea, or no more than two to four cans of caffeinated sodas) in patients with hypertension. Likewise, such drinks should be avoided for at least one hour before blood pressure is measured so that an accurate reading, uninfluenced by caffeine, can be obtained.

Although some studies have reported that excess coffee consumption may cause some elevation of "bad" cholesterol (low-density lipoprotein, or LDL) and triglycerides in the blood, the evidence is not compelling. Any slight changes are probably of no importance. In fact, after a tolerance to caffeine develops, caffeinated drinks have no effect on blood pressure or heart rate.

Finally, one study has reported that men consuming large quantities of tea, which contains antioxidants, have a reduced risk of heart attack (see Question 96). It is noteworthy that coffee also contains antioxidants and, surprisingly, soluble fiber, both of which may be beneficial.

57 Is It Safe to Take Estrogen Before and after Menopause if You Have Hypertension?

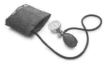

When they were initially introduced, oral contraceptives ("the pill") contained relatively high concentrations of two female hormones, estrogen and progesterone. Such high hormone concentrations may possibly cause salt retention and an increased blood volume, as well as other changes that result in the constriction of arterioles with an elevation of blood pressure (BP); however, the exact cause of the elevated BP remains unclear. With the original oral contraceptives, 5 to 18 percent of the women taking them developed some elevation of BP. Fortunately, their BP returned to its original levels after discontinuing the medication. Rarely, the high doses of estrogens and progesterone in the original oral contraceptives were associated with blood clots and strokes. In men, high concentrations of estrogen can also increase the risk of cardiovascular disease such as heart attack and stroke.

> *Oral estrogens (especially if taken in high doses) may increase blood pressure, although, if taken through the skin by patch, blood pressure may remain unchanged or be reduced.*

Since then, the concentrations of estrogen and progesterone in the pill have been considerably reduced. Today, oral contraceptives rarely increase BP. Estrogens taken alone and in very high doses may increase BP, but low doses do not bring about hypertension and may actually reduce BP. This is another situation in which more is not necessarily better.

The effectiveness of estrogen replacement therapy (ERT) in low dosage, administered as a pill or skin patch, was reported in two circumstances:

- in the treatment of osteoporosis
- in controlling menopausal symptoms such as hot flashes and vaginal dryness

A number of studies indicate that estrogens decrease the risk of heart disease. The explanation for the lower risk of heart and blood vessel disease and stroke in premenopausal women compared to men of similar age probably stems from the fact that premenopausal women have lower BP and lower levels of "bad" cholesterol (LDL—low-density lipoprotein) and higher levels of "good" cholesterol (HDL—high-density lipoprotein) than men. These favorable cholesterol levels are likely related to the high levels of estrogen in premenopausal women. After menopause, women lose these cardiovascular protective factors due to the marked reduction of estrogen in their circulation. As a result, their risk of cardiovascular disease becomes equal to or even greater than that in men of the same age. A three-year study of 875 postmenopausal women by the National Institutes of Health revealed that ERT decreased LDL by about 20 percent, increased HDL, elevated BP, and did not increase the occurrence of cancers. Nevertheless, it is important to recognize that the incidence of cancer of the uterus may be doubled in postmenopausal women taking ERT without progesterone as compared with postmenopausal women not using estrogen. Whether estrogen increases the incidence of breast cancer in postmenopausal women remains controversial.

More recently, a rise in systolic BP has been reported in postmenopausal women taking oral estrogen; however, if the estrogen is delivered through the skin from a patch, the BP remains unchanged or is even lower in postmenopausal women. It is advised that oral estrogen and oral contraceptives be avoided in hypertensive premenopausal or postmenopausal women, especially if the BP is not well controlled.

In deciding who to treat with ERT, a physician must talk with the patient, weighing the value of the treatment against the possible risk. ERT may be necessary to control menopausal symptoms and vaginal dryness. However, even a low concentration of estrogen should not be given to men, since it does not appear to protect them from cardiovascular disease and furthermore may cause impotence and breast enlargement. Previously, if post-menopausal women had osteoporosis (detected by bone density testing or a history suggesting bone fractures due to fragile bones), ERT used to be employed commonly along with calcium and vitamin D supplements and a recommendation of appropriate exercise. With the advent of nonhormonal approaches to osteoporosis, such as bisphosphonates (Fosamax, Actonel, Boniva, and Reclast), there has been a decided movement away from using estrogens, and they are no longer considered to be first-line agents for the treatment of postmenopausal osteoporosis. Rather, agents like the bisphosphonates, which prevent bone loss, dominate the therapeutic landscape for the treatment of postmenopausal osteoporosis. They do not affect the blood pressure.

In patients who are to be treated with ERT for menopausal symptoms of estrogen deficiency, progesterone should be used with the estrogen to protect patients from the possibility of developing uterine cancer. (Progesterone counteracts the stimulatory effects of estrogen on the lining of the uterus and thus reduces the chance of uterine cancer.) It is noteworthy that the combination of estrogen and progesterone can slightly increase the chance of blood clots and gallbladder disease. Of course, if a hysterectomy has been performed previously, progesterone need not be added. Finally, ERT is not recommended in patients who have had breast cancer or who have a family history of breast cancer.

58 What Is Preeclampsia (Toxemia of Pregnancy)? Does Hypertension Increase My Chances of Getting It, and How Should It Be Treated?

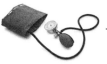

Preeclampsia occurs in approximately 3 percent of all pregnancies, most often during the first pregnancy. It is usually characterized by hypertension, retention of water and salt (manifested by swelling of the ankles, face, and hands, plus weight gain), and increased protein in the urine in the third trimester of pregnancy. This condition was originally called toxemia of pregnancy, because it was thought to result from a toxin that appeared in the circulation after the twentieth week of pregnancy. Today, however, physicians consider the cause of the condition to be a mystery.

Normally during the first and second trimester of a pregnancy, a woman's diastolic blood pressure (BP) decreases approximately 5 to 10 mm Hg, with little change in systolic pressure. In the third trimester, the diastolic pressure returns to its initial level.

Preeclampsia occurs most frequently in the following types of women:

• young women (in their teens) or women older than forty years of age during their first pregnancy

• women with a family history of preeclampsia

• women carrying multiple fetuses

• African-American women

• women with preexisting hypertension, diabetes, kidney disease, or obesity

• women who had preeclampsia with a former pregnancy

Recognizing preeclampsia and treating it appropriately are extremely important to prevent the development of a very serious condition known as eclampsia. This latter condition occurs in about 1 in 1,500 pregnancies and is associated with pronounced hypertension, severe headaches, visual disturbances, abdominal pains, seizures, unconsciousness, and even death of the mother and fetus.

The presence of high BP before pregnancy should not deter you from becoming pregnant, as your pregnancy may be completely normal (see Question 59). Nevertheless, because the presence of hypertension increases the risk of preeclampsia, BP should be carefully monitored in hypertensive women who are pregnant, and appropriate medication should continue to be administered. Aldomet (alpha-methyldopa) has been used successfully for many years and has proven safe for both mother and fetus. Beta blockers, labetalol, and the vasodilator Apresoline (hydralazine) also appear effective and safe, and diuretics ("water pills") may occasionally be indicated. Other antihypertensive medications should usually be discontinued and avoided during pregnancy, especially ACE inhibitors, angiotensin receptor blockers, and direct renin inhibitors, because they may hurt the fetus, retarding growth and causing birth defects or even death. In patients with preeclampsia, the drugs mentioned above (with the exception of diuretics) can be used, bed rest is sometimes indicated (to lower BP and to improve blood flow to the fetus), and hospitalization may be required. Early delivery by cesarean section will rapidly resolve the symptoms and signs of severe preeclampsia, prevent the development of eclampsia, and usually return the mother's BP to the level it was before the onset of pregnancy.

> *The presence of high blood pressure before pregnancy should not deter you from becoming pregnant, as your pregnancy may be completely normal.*

Close monitoring of the BP should be continued after delivery, since preeclampsia may occasionally appear at that time. If the BP remains elevated for six weeks after delivery, further investigation for another cause of the hypertension is indicated. It should be emphasized that women with hypertension or other risks for preeclampsia who are planning to become pregnant should be monitored closely by physicians who have expertise in managing hypertension.

59 If I Have Hypertension, Should I Avoid Getting Pregnant?

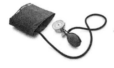

Hypertensive women do not necessarily have to avoid pregnancy. It is a good sign if you have had a previous uncomplicated pregnancy. If your hypertension is not severe, you have a very good chance of carrying a pregnancy to term without a problem. You should, however, be under the supervision of an obstetrician from the very outset of the pregnancy. If you are taking an ACE inhibitor, an angiotensin receptor blocker (ARB), or a direct renin inhibitor (see Question 58) for your hypertension, you should stop using the medication before you become pregnant or as soon as you know you are pregnant, because these drugs may cause fetal damage or mortality. If you have hypertension that is not controlled by lifestyle changes and/or medication, you should consult your physician and an obstetrician before becoming pregnant. If you become pregnant and then discover that you have hypertension, you should immediately consult a physician and an obstetrician.

60 Should I Limit My Activities if I Have Hypertension?

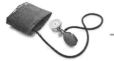

You should limit your activities only if you have already experienced complications — such as heart disease, kidney disease, or stroke — from hypertension. In general, aerobic exercise (running, walking, jogging, swimming, and so on) is beneficial for hypertension, because it may lower blood pressure, improve cardiovascular fitness, and help in reducing excess weight. For patients with uncomplicated hypertension (having no target-organ damage), there is no benefit from restricting activities or cutting back on your workload. If negative complications such as heart disease, kidney disease, or stroke have already occurred, your physician will advise you about limiting your activities. Typically, the physician may recommend a supervised, graded exercise program.

Many doctors believe that it is prudent for most people over forty-five to obtain a stress test before embarking on any exercise program. The test records the electrical activity of your heart while you are exercising on a treadmill. This information is very helpful in determining any abnormalities of the blood supply to the heart, which might make strenuous exercise inadvisable.

61 Is the Hypertension That Sometimes Occurs with Sleep Apnea Serious, and How Is It Treated?

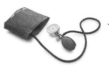

Sleep apnea is a periodic cessation of breathing during sleep (see Question 38). It usually lasts anywhere from 20 seconds to 3 minutes and may occur from 10 to 15 times per hour. This sleep disorder affects 2 to 4 percent of middle-aged women and men. Two types of sleep apnea are recognized: that caused by airway obstruction in the pharyngeal area, and that caused by decreased activity of the nerve impulses that drive the respiratory muscles.

Airway obstruction in the pharyngeal area (back of the mouth and upper airway tube) may result from anatomical disturbances in the back of the mouth or tongue with "pharyngeal crowding." Obesity often contributes to the problem, and alcohol consumption can aggravate it. Loud snoring is extremely common — often associated with choking or gasping and the cessation of breathing — and is frequently witnessed by the bed partner or someone else. Chronic sleepiness during the day, intellectual deterioration, personality changes, behavioral disorders, memory loss, and impotence may occur. Furthermore, episodes of apnea may be accompanied by a slowing down or speeding up of the heart rate, the development of hypertension, incidents of stroke or heart attack, and premature death.

> *Episodes of obstructive sleep apnea may be accompanied by a slowing down or speeding up of the heart rate, the development of hypertension, incidents of stroke or heart attack, and premature death.*

The diagnosis of this type of sleep apnea can be confirmed by an overnight sleep study with appropriate recordings to determine brain waves, muscle activity, and oxygen deficiency. Treatment consists of weight reduction (if indicated), the avoidance of alcohol, the avoidance of sleeping in the supine position (on the back), the use of oral devices to keep the airway open at night, and the use of a pressure apparatus to deliver air continuously to the patient at night (called a CPAP machine). Surgical procedures to ameliorate the obstructed airflow may occasionally be necessary. If the episodes of hypertension are modest and only occur with the apnea, antihypertensive medication is probably not indicated. On the other hand, if the patient already has hypertension and a marked rise in blood pressure occurs during apnea, it is important that blood pressure be controlled with antihypertensive medication.

The second type of sleep apnea results from a *decreased activity of the nerve impulses that drive the respiratory muscles.* Obesity and hypertension are less prominent with this disorder. Other manifestations are similar to patients with obstructive sleep apnea, although an overnight sleep study will reveal recurrent apneas that are not accompanied by respiratory effort. In individuals with this condition, carbon dioxide in the blood tends to progressively increase during the night. Some patients benefit from continuous air delivery with a pressure apparatus and from the additional delivery of oxygen, if needed.

62 If I Have Diabetes Mellitus, Does That Increase My Chances of Suffering from Disease Complications Related to Hypertension?

Diabetes mellitus is definitely linked to a greater risk of developing complications related to hypertension. The combination of diabetes and hypertension increases the chance of premature heart attacks, strokes, and kidney failure (see Question 43). We recommend that diabetic/hypertensive patients receive intensive treatment for both conditions. In these patients, the goal of treatment for hypertension should be to reduce blood pressure to less than 130/80 mm Hg. Excellent control of blood sugar is also helpful in this situation.

63 Will Antihypertensive Drugs Interfere with My Physical or Mental Activity and Be a Danger to My Health?

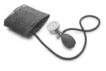

Very rarely will antihypertensive drugs interfere with mental function or physical activity, and they should never be a danger to your health when properly administered. Remember, it is always better to treat hypertension than to leave it untreated. Nevertheless, some medications should not be used in patients who require maximal physical performance or who compete in amateur and professional athletic events. Furthermore, some antihypertensive agents (e.g., clonidine, methyldopa, reserpine, guanethidine, guanabenz, guanadrel) may cause fatigue and impair mental alertness, which could pose a hazard when driving a vehicle, flying a plane, or working with dangerous machinery.

> *Beta blockers slow the heart rate, can slightly decrease exercise tolerance, and, although rarely, may cause fatigue; they are therefore a poor choice for anyone engaging in strenuous sports.*

Beta blockers slow the heart rate, can slightly decrease exercise tolerance, and, although rarely, may cause fatigue; they are therefore a poor choice for anyone engaging in strenuous sports. These drugs may also cause bronchospasm in patients with asthma, which could further compromise exercise enjoyment and athletic performance. Depression has occasionally been observed with some beta blockers (those that reach the brain). In a small percentage of men, such agents may lead to impotence and a loss of sexual desire, which can further aggravate depression. Long-acting diuretics were reported to cause impotence in a small percentage of men; however, recent observations do not indicate that diuretics cause impotence (see Question 66).

If beta blockers are discontinued in patients with evidence of coronary artery disease, the dosage should be decreased gradually over a number of days. The gradual weaning is necessary to avoid any risk of heart attack.

Clonidine (Catapres) acts on the central nervous system and lowers blood pressure (BP) by decreasing the activity of the sympathetic nervous system, thereby permitting the arterioles to dilate and the BP to decrease. In large doses it can induce extreme fatigue, drowsiness, and sedation. Impaired thinking, psychological problems, and depression have been observed, and impotence may occur. Weakness and unsteadiness affect approximately 6 percent of patients using this medication. Certainly, this drug should not be given to patients requiring alertness, normal reflex reaction time, and skillful coordination. Another concern with patients consuming sizable doses of clonidine is that this medication should never be stopped abruptly, as sudden termination may result in a very marked and potentially dangerous elevation of BP.

Any antihypertensive drug can potentially lower BP excessively and cause a feeling of faintness and unsteadiness, which could even result in a loss of consciousness and a fall with possible serious injury. Patients vary considerably in their BP response to the various antihypertensive medications. Therefore, it is reasonable and prudent to start with relatively low doses of these drugs and to check the BP of patients in both seated and standing positions. If a marked decrease of BP occurs when a patient stands up — a condition sometimes associated with faintness — then a smaller dose of the medication is indicated.

In a small percentage of patients, the alpha$_1$-blocking drugs (mainly Doxazosin) are likely to cause a pronounced drop in BP when standing within a short time after the first dose is taken. For this reason, the first dose should be taken at bedtime rather than during the day, as having a recumbent position in bed will prevent the loss of consciousness that might occur in the standing position. Fortunately, after this possible first-dose effect, alpha$_1$ blockers can be used without fear of subsequent hypotensive episodes. However, careful monitoring of the BP is indicated as this medication is increased.

In general, when low or moderate doses of antihypertensive drugs are used, or when combinations of low or moderate doses of such drugs are used to control BP, there are relatively few bothersome side effects.

64 What Is a Hypertensive Emergency?

In a hypertensive emergency, the patient is at risk for developing severe damage in the target organs (heart, brain, kidneys); these negative hypertensive complications can be prevented or minimized by intensive treatment of the high blood pressure, sometimes with medications given by injection into a muscle or a vein. Common hypertensive emergencies include heart failure with fluid in the lungs, signs of impending stroke, and evidence of kidney failure as determined by urinalysis and blood tests. Even mild hypertension is an emergency in the presence of heart failure or a dissecting aneurysm that may rupture and hemorrhage. The typical hypertensive emergency is "hypertensive encephalopathy," a condition in which the brain swells because of very high blood pressure, leading to severe headache, intermittent blindness, nausea, vomiting, and confusion.

> *In a hypertensive emergency, high blood pressure is leading to damage in the target organs (heart, brain, kidneys), which can be prevented or minimized by intensive treatment of the high blood pressure.*

The goal of treatment is to reduce blood pressure to nearly normal levels within three to four hours by giving blood pressure-lowering medications by injection. Oral medications should not be used since they are less reliable in controlling hypertensive emergencies. Hypertensive emergencies should not occur if high blood pressure is treated appropriately and effectively. In fact, hypertensive encephalopathy has been seen only rarely since effective treatment of hypertension became available. When it does occur, it usually affects patients who have not had their hypertension treated or who have discontinued treatment.

65 When Are Medications Indicated for the Treatment of Hypertension?

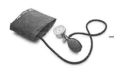

Stroke, heart attack, heart and kidney failure, and hardening of the arteries — all of these occur least frequently when blood pressures (BPs) remain at 135/85 mm Hg or less. Establishing an accurate, average BP level is therefore essential before starting treatment. It is important to determine whether an elevated BP obtained in the doctor's office might be due to anxiety ("white-coat hypertension"). In this endeavor, having the patient, a family member, or friend record the BP at home can be very helpful in determining a truly accurate pressure (see Questions 14 and 19). When taking BP measurements, the patient should be in a seated position and remain relaxed in a quiet environment for at least five minutes before the pressure is recorded, and the BP cuff should be the right size and placed on the arm at about the level of the sternum (breastbone). Cigarette smoking, the consumption of drinks containing caffeine, and exercise should be avoided for approximately one hour before the BP is measured. If the BP is only slightly elevated, lifestyle changes (such as reducing weight, limiting salt and alcohol intake, getting adequate exercise, and consuming a potassium-rich, low-fat diet) may reduce pressure into normal ranges. Although it is doubtful that cigarette smoking contributes to the development of hypertension, the cessation of smoking is still extremely important — there is no more serious health risk for heart and blood vessel disease, cancer, obstructive lung disease, and emphysema. Furthermore, smoking enhances a person's risks of developing the negative complications related to hypertension (see Question 51).

If, despite lifestyle changes, elevations of blood pressure (more that 140/90 mm Hg but less than 160/100 mm Hg) persist for three to six months, antihypertensive medication should be started.

If, despite lifestyle changes, elevations of blood pressure (more than 140/90 mm Hg) persist for three to six months, antihypertensive medication should be started.

It is noteworthy that elevated systolic pressure poses more of a risk for negative complications of hypertension than diastolic pressure elevations do (see Question 20). Therefore, even if only systolic pressures are elevated, treatment to normalize the pressure is indicated. With a BP of 160/100 mm Hg or greater, lifestyle changes and antihypertensive medications should be started immediately. Even if pressures only vary from 140/90 mm Hg to less than 160/90 mm Hg, intensive treatment with drugs and diet to lower BP should be instituted if the patient has any evidence of heart, kidney, brain, or vascular disease. Only very rarely is hospitalization required to initiate very intensive treatment (for example, when hypertension is very severe and/or accompanied by acute damage to the brain, heart, kidneys, and blood vessels).

66 What Drugs Are Available for Treating Hypertension? How Do They Work, and What Are Their Side Effects? Are Generic Medications as Good as Brand-Name Drugs?

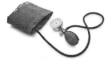

Although the choice of antihypertensive drugs depends somewhat on age, gender, race, accompanying diseases, and medical history, the main objective of treatment is to normalize blood pressure (BP) and to prevent and/or reduce damage to the brain, heart, kidneys, and blood vessels. The final decision regarding the choice of medications should be left to your doctor, who knows you best. Appropriate lifestyle changes should always be initiated; they will usually have a beneficial effect on the patient's health as well as lower BP and often result in reducing the amount of medication needed for BP control.

The commonly used oral antihypertensive medications include diuretics, beta blockers, ACE inhibitors, angiotensin receptor blockers, direct renin inhibitors, calcium-channel blockers, and alpha₁ blockers.

Currently, more than 135 single antihypertensive medications are commercially available in the United States, as well as another 50 to 60 fixed-dose combinations of two drugs. The commonly used oral antihypertensive medications (those taken by mouth) include diuretics, beta blockers, ACE inhibitors, angiotensin receptor blockers, direct renin inhibitors, calcium-channel blockers, and alpha$_1$ blockers. Combinations of a diuretic with a potassium-conserving agent, a beta blocker, an ACE inhibitor, or an angiotensin receptor blocker are also popular therapeutic options. Less commonly used antihypertensives include agents that lower BP by depressing sympathetic nerve activity (a part of your nervous system that, when active, constricts the arterioles), thereby dilating the arterioles. Table 8 (see next page) lists most of the antihypertensives available in the United States and their mechanisms of action.

Combinations may be more convenient when the patient must take a large number of pills each day. Nevertheless, some physicians prefer to determine how individual drugs affect the patient before using them in combination, as one of the drugs used as a single-agent therapy may adequately control the patient's BP. Furthermore, if undesirable side effects occur, it is often not possible to tell which drug in a combination is responsible. However, the current trend is to start with combination tablets, and this may partly be because combination drugs are sometimes less expensive than two drugs purchased individually.

Long-acting diuretics (thiazides and thiazidelike drugs) — also known as "water pills" — have a duration of action of approximately twenty four hours. They are highly effective, safe drugs with which to initiate treatment of hypertension. Their action on the kidney tubules eliminates salt and water and causes the arteries to relax, thereby reducing BP. Dietary salt should be limited when these agents are prescribed, because limiting salt consumption enhances the antihypertensive effect and may reduce the amount of diuretic required to reduce BP. African Americans, older patients, and obese individuals are often salt sensitive; diuretics are particularly effective in the treatment of these individuals.

Table 8. Brand and Generic Names of Some Antihypertensive Drugs Commonly Used in the United States

Diuretics (cause excretion of salt and water; dilate blood vessels)	Long-acting thiazide diuretics (act on distal tubules in kidneys)
	Diuril/Enduron/Esidrix (hydrochlorothiazide), Hygroton (chlorthalidone), Lozol (indapamide), Metolazone (myrox, zaroxolyn), Naqua (trichlormethiazide), Thalitone (chlorthalidone)
	Short-acting diuretics (act on loop tubules in kidneys)
	Bumex (bumetanide), Demadex (torsemide), Edecrin (ethacrynic acid), Lasix (furosemide)
	Potassium-sparing diuretics (weak diuretics cause kidneys to retain potassium)
	Aldactone (spironolactone), Dyrenium (triamterene), Inspira (eplerenone), Midamor (amiloride)
Beta blockers (diminish effect of norepinephrine and epinephrine on heart and blood vessels)	Blocadren (timolol), Corgard (nadolol), Inderal, Inderal LA (propranolol), Tenormin (atenolol), Lopressor/Toprol-XL (metoprolol)
Vasodilating beta blockers	Bystolic (nebivolol), Coreg (carvedilol), Trandate/Normodyne (labetalol)
ACE inhibitors (prevent production of angiotensin)	Accupril (quinapril), Altace (ramipril), Capoten (captopril), Lotensin (benazepril), Mavik (trandolapril), Monopril (fosinopril), Prinivil, Zestril (lisinopril), Univasc (moexipril), Vasotec (enalapril)
Direct renin inhibitors (prevent production of angiotensin and block renin elevations caused by ACE inhibitors and angiotensin receptor blockers)	Aliskirin (tekturna)

(cont'd.)

Table 8. Brand and Generic Names of Some Antihypertensive Drugs Commonly Used in the United States (cont'd.)

Angiotensin blockers (block the effect of angiotensin on receptors of this hormone in blood vessels and the adrenal gland)	Atacand (candesartan), Avapro (irbesartan), Cozaar (losartan), Diovan (valsartan), Micardis (telmisartan), Benicar (olmesartan), Teveten (eprosartan)
Calcium-channel blockers (long acting) (block entry of calcium into heart or blood vessel cells)	*Nondihydropyridines (cause vasodilation and slow electrical condition of the heart)*
	Cardizem CD/Cardizem SR/Tiazac (diltiazem), Dilacor XL/Isoptin SR/Calan SR/Verelan, Covera HS (verapamil)
	Dihydropyridines (cause only dilation of arteries and no effect on heart)
	Adalat CC (nifedipine), Cardene XL (nicardipine), DynaCirc/DynaCirc CR (isradipine), Norvasc (amlodipine), Plendil (felodipine), Procardia XL/Adolat CC (nifedipine), Sular (nisoldipine)
Alpha₁ blockers (diminish the constricting action of norepinephrine and epinephrine on blood vessels)	Cardura [long acting] (doxazosin), Hytrin [long acting] (terazosin), Minipress [short acting] (prazosin)
Alpha₂ agonists (cause depression of the sympathetic nervous system, which results in vasodilation)	Aldomet (methyldopa), Catapres (clonidine), Tenex (guanfacine), Wytensin (guanabenz)
Adrenergic depleters (diminish norepinephrine in sympathetic nerves, which results in vasodilation)	Hylorel (guanadrel), Ismelin (guanethidine), Reserpine (serpasil)
Vasodilators (cause vasodilation by directly causing muscles in the vessels to relax)	Apresoline (hydralazine), Loniten (minoxidil)

Increased urination occurs when long-acting diuretics are initially taken, but it should not be a long-term problem unless the patient has significant prostatic obstruction. Although these drugs are associated with few side effects, there is no strong evidence that males experience impotence. Occasionally, the level of potassium in the blood decreases significantly, which may alter the rhythm of the heart. The lower doses of diuretics now used routinely ensure that the problem of low blood potassium is a rare one. In addition, low-potassium problems can be prevented by consuming potassium-rich foods and/or prescribing potassium tablets or a potassium-conserving agent combined with the thiazide. Gout may be precipitated by diuretics, so these drugs should be used cautiously if the patient has a history of gout.

Loop diuretics affect a different part of the kidney tubule than that targeted by long-acting diuretics. In addition, they are more potent and have a more rapid onset of action than thiazides. Lasix (furosemide) is a short-acting (four to six hours) drug that is indicated if the patient has severely impaired kidney function or heart failure; it is more effective in eliminating salt and water than are the long-acting diuretics. Loop diuretics must be taken twice daily, and they do not decrease the BP as effectively as the thiazides.

Beta blockers are antihypertensive agents that block two hormones — norepinephrine (released from the sympathetic nervous system) and epinephrine (released from adrenal glands) — from reaching their receptors in the heart. In this way, these blockers reduce heart rate and its pumping force, and some diminish resistance (constriction) in arterioles. In addition, beta blockers suppress production of renin in the kidney, thereby preventing the formation of angiotensin (a powerful constrictor of arteries). As a result of all these actions, the BP decreases.

Beta blockers provide another benefit by reducing the work of the heart and its oxygen requirement in patients who have angina (pain or a pressure sensation in the chest due to a deficient oxygen supply to the heart). Such drugs can help control rapid and irregular heart rhythm, and they have been shown to reduce the chance of a second heart attack. In addition, beta blockers may be beneficial in treating heart failure.

Beta blockers must be administered cautiously, however, as sometimes they may worsen heart failure and may impair electrical conduction in the heart. Because blocking beta receptors in the lung can cause bronchial constriction, these drugs may precipitate or aggravate asthma attacks. They can also be associated with fatigue, decreased exercise tolerance, and cold hands, and some users may experience impotence and decreased sexual drive. However, most individuals experience few of these side effects. A slight increase in blood sugar and blood fats (triglycerides) and a decrease in "good" cholesterol (HDL) may occur. In patients receiving insulin, beta blockers may mask the symptoms of low blood sugar. Some beta blockers mainly affect the heart, whereas others have a more generalized effect and reach the brain, where they may cause depression.

ACE (angiotensin-converting enzyme) inhibitors restrain the formation of angiotensin, a powerful constrictor of arteries. These drugs also permit a buildup of bradykinin, a substance that causes blood vessels to dilate. The end result is a lower BP. ACE inhibitors are not only effective as antihypertensive drugs, they are also very valuable in treating some types of heart failure, especially if the disease is caused by hypertension, and in slowing the progression of kidney failure in diabetics. With severe kidney failure, however, ACE inhibitors or angiotensin receptor blockers may aggravate the failure and cause retention of potassium. In general, physicians avoid potassium-sparing drugs and potassium supplementation in patients taking ACE inhibitors or angiotensin receptor blockers.

Approximately 10 to 20 percent of all people who take these drugs develop a dry, hacking cough, which may require them to discontinue taking it. Rarely, the drugs may cause a skin rash or diminish one's sense of taste; very rarely, an acute allergic reaction (anaphylaxis) is accompanied by swelling of the tongue, face, and other tissues (angioedema), and a marked drop in blood pressure, which may be fatal. ACE inhibitors should not be used during pregnancy or if pregnancy is anticipated, because they may cause serious birth defects and fetal death.

Angiotensin receptor blockers (ARBs) inhibit the effects of angiotensin, thereby preventing the constriction of blood vessels; as a consequence, BP is lowered. Unlike ACE inhibitors, these drugs do not cause an increase in bradykinin, and they don't produce a dry cough or angioedema. Allergic reactions and side effects are very rare. Like ACE inhibitors, angiotensin inhibitors should be avoided during pregnancy or if pregnancy is planned. If potassium is elevated in the blood, these drugs should be avoided.

Calcium-channel blockers consist of two types:

- the dihydropyridines, which cause blood vessels to dilate

- the nondihydropyridines, which cause blood vessel dilation but also slow down electrical conduction in the heart

Both types of these drugs exert their effects by blocking calcium channels and thus diminishing access of calcium to the smooth muscles of the blood vessels. In addition, the nondihydropyridines diminish access of calcium to the muscles of the heart. BP is lowered by the vasodilation, which also increases blood supply to the heart and can be helpful in treating patients with angina (pain or a pressure sensation in the chest from a diminished flow of blood and oxygen to the heart). Likewise, calcium-channel blockers may benefit individuals with narrowed arteries in the legs, and they are particularly effective in elderly patients and individuals with systolic hypertension. Because they slow electrical conduction in the heart, the nondihydropyridines can be effective in the treatment of some heart irregularities, but they should not be used when electrical conduction in the heart is impaired, heart failure is present, or the patient is already taking beta blockers. Some nondihydropyridine calcium-channel blockers may be indicated in patients following a heart attack, if beta blockers cannot be used. Beta blockers and nondihydropyridines should not be used together.

Side effects of calcium-channel blockers include constipation (only nondihydropyridines), swelling of the lower legs and feet, headaches, swollen gums, rash, and rapid heartbeat (only dihydropyridines). Consumption of grapefruit juice can impair the liver's ability to metabolize and eliminate some of these drugs, so this juice should not be consumed two hours before or two hours after taking calcium-channel blockers, as they may accumulate in the body and become toxic.

Alpha$_1$ blockers inhibit the effect of norepinephrine, a hormone that is released from the sympathetic nerves. Since norepinephrine normally constricts arteries, blocking its action causes the arteries to dilate and thus reduces BP. Alpha$_1$ blockers may improve urinary flow in men with partial urinary obstruction due to an enlarged prostate. In addition, they may increase "good" cholesterol (HDL) in blood and modestly lower total cholesterol and triglycerides. Rarely, the first dose may cause a pronounced drop in blood pressure, accompanied by dizziness or fainting on standing. This effect is usually not a problem if the first dose is taken at bedtime, when the patient is recumbent, or if a small dose is given initially. Other side effects include headaches, nasal congestion, dry mouth, and, rarely, urinary incontinence in women.

Alpha$_2$ agonists exert their effects in the brain and diminish the activity of the sympathetic nerves to the arteries and heart. As a result, the smooth muscles in the arteries relax and dilate. The heart rate does not increase, however, and the BP is reduced. These drugs are not used very often because of their potential side effects — sedation, drowsiness, decreased alertness, and fatigue —

which may significantly disrupt mental and physical performance. Nevertheless, they may be beneficial in patients experiencing panic attacks or symptoms of withdrawal from alcohol or drug addiction.

The alpha$_2$ agonist clonidine (Catapres) can be applied to the skin in a patch, which is effective for one week, and it appears to cause fewer side effects than when it is taken as a pill. The "dry mouth" effect produced by some of these drugs can be particularly annoying. In addition, these antihypertensive agents may cause impotence and mental depression. Alpha-methyldopa (Aldomet) is a popular option for patients who are pregnant because of its safety and efficacy.

Stopping the use of some alpha$_2$ agonists abruptly may cause the BP to increase rapidly to very high levels — high enough to cause a stroke. Therefore, physician consultation about the drug and a gradual tapering off of the drug are important when its use is discontinued.

Vasodilating beta blockers include Normodyne, Trandate, Bystolic, and Coreg. These drugs lower BP by decreasing the constriction of arteries but have little effect on the heart rate and the pumping force of the heart.

On rare occasions, these drugs may cause a pronounced drop in BP on standing, an effect that is most likely to occur at the beginning of treatment and when taking large doses. These drugs may also cause a failure to ejaculate, asthmalike breathing, itching of the scalp, skin eruptions, and — only rarely — severe liver damage.

Adrenergic depleters cause a depletion in the sympathetic nerves of norepinephrine (the hormone released from these nerves). By so doing, they cause arteries to dilate, thereby decreasing BP. Today most of these drugs are not available because of their side effects (reserpine may cause gastric ulceration and mental depression; Ismelin (guanethidine) and Hylorel (guanadrel) sometimes caused a pronounced drop in BP on standing, ejaculation failure, fluid retention, and diarrhea, and their use has been discontinued. Indeed, many more acceptable drugs for the treatment of hypertension are available, but reserpine may occasionally be used.

Vasodilators act directly on the muscles in the walls of arteries, causing them to dilate and thereby reducing blood pressure. These powerful dilators of the arteries are often used in patients who do not respond to other antihypertensive medications.

Minoxidil (Loniten) is more potent than hydralazine (Apresoline) and is especially valuable in the therapy of severe hypertension accompanied by impairment of kidney function. Loniten can lead to the retention of salt and water, so this agent must be used in combination with powerful diuretics (water pills). Hydralazine may cause a rapid heart rate, which may aggravate pain or pressure sensations in the chest (angina); therefore, beta blockers are often employed along with this drug to slow the heart rate and prevent angina. Other potential side effects include flushing and headaches. Hydralazine can also rarely cause a connective tissue disease similar to lupus (which usually subsides on discontinuation of the drug), and minoxidil, even in low doses, causes hair growth over the entire body in about 80 percent of patients, which is a serious problem for women.

Some antihypertensive drugs are available only as brand-name versions, because pharmaceutical companies that originally develop drugs have seventeen years before their patent rights expire and hence generic versions can be marketed. The generic drugs that are available should be identical in activity and side effects to their brand-name predecessors. You can be sure they have been carefully tested and evaluated by the Food and Drug Administration. Thus, there is no reason to avoid using the cheaper generic-named antihypertensive medications when they are available.

There are currently a great number of combination drugs (e.g., an alpha and a beta blocker, a diuretic and a beta blockers, a diuretic and angiotensin receptor antagonist, a potassium-sparing drug and a thiazide diuretic, a calcium antagonist). The question arises, "Should I take a tablet with a combination of two or more antihypertensive drugs? Such combinations are becoming increasingly popular, and pharmaceutical companies want to increase the use of their patent-protected drug with another drug that is generic, in particular a low dose of a diuretic.

There may be advantages to using such combinations. Their use may improve patients' adherence to therapy and reduce the cost of their medications. The combination may increase the potency of their antihypertensive regimen, and less than a full dose of both drugs may be administered to achieve a BP goal. However, there are also disadvantages that cause many physicians not to use such combinations. These include an inability to know which drug is responsible for side effects, if they occur, and a restriction of the ability to change the dose of one of the drugs without altering the dose of the other.

Initially, then, many physicians prefer to use individual drugs rather than combination of drugs. However, if the BP is well controlled with several different drugs, it may be desirable to use a combination of two drugs if the individual dosage of each drug remains the same and if the cost is similar or less when a combination is used.

A combination of an antihypertensive drug with a drug that lowers cholesterol may be used to control BP and harmful (LDL) cholesterol levels. However, for the reasons stated above, many physicians prefer to initiate treatment with individual drugs rather than a combination.

67 What Are the Newest Drugs for the Treatment of Hypertension, and How Do They Work? Should I Switch to These Medications?

The only new type of antihypertensive drug recently marketed is the direct renin inhibitor aliskirin (Tekturna), which acts in a different manner than the angiotensin receptor blockers but provides the same effect on the blood pressure and a similar absence of side effects.

"Newer" does not necessarily mean "better" when it comes to antihypertensive medications. Some older drugs have excellent track records for successfully controlling blood pressure and preventing disease complications related to hypertension, cause few if any side effects, and are relatively inexpensive. *If your blood pressure is under good control and you are experiencing no side effects, you should continue with your current medication.* Any decision to change medication should be made in consultation with your physician.

68 Are the Newer Antihypertensive Medications Better Than the Old Ones?

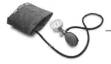

Clinical trials comparing newer medications to the older ones have not demonstrated any convincing evidence for the superiority of the newer drugs in lowering blood pressure. In general, the newcomers appear no more effective in reducing blood pressure than the older ones, nor are they more effective in reducing the disease complications of hypertension. The exceptions are the ACE inhibitor drugs and angiotensin receptor blockers (ARBs), which have shown superior benefits in diabetic patients who have protein (albumin) in the urine and in patients with heart failure due to elevated blood pressure. ACE inhibitors and ARBs can improve blood flow in the kidneys, reduce protein in the urine, and prevent the progression of kidney disease. They also reduce the workload on a failing heart. On the other hand, the beta blockers (an older class of antihypertensive drugs) are the most effective drugs in preventing recurrent heart attacks in hypertensive patients as well as in patients who have normal blood pressure. Some beta blockers have been shown to reduce migraine

> *Newer medications have not demonstrated any convincing superiority relative to older antihypertensive drugs in lowering blood pressure.*

headaches and may be the drug of choice for hypertensive patients who have this symptom.

69 What Medications Will My Doctor Prescribe for My Hypertension? When Are Certain Drugs Indicated or to Be Avoided (Contraindicated)?

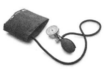

Most specialists who treat hypertension agree with the guidelines proposed by the *Report of the Joint National Committee on Prevention, Detection, Evaluation, and Treatment of High Blood Pressure* (*JNC7* report). The committee behind this report, which meets periodically as part of the National High Blood Pressure Education Program, is composed of approximately forty-five prestigious organizations that have an interest and expertise in the management of hypertension. The recommendations of this committee are very logical and reasonable, because they are based on the latest scientific information coupled with years of experience with most of the antihypertensive drugs.

As noted, "newer" does not necessarily mean "better" when it comes to antihypertensive drugs. It should be appreciated that diuretics have the longest track record in treating hypertension, and their ability to decrease the disease complications associated with hypertension and mortality from hypertension has been established by many carefully controlled studies. A long-acting thiazide diuretic (water pill) may be recommended by your physician as initial therapy if no good medical reasons exist not to use this type of drug. This recommendation holds true for the vast majority of patients with stage 1 hypertension; that is, with blood pressure (BP) less than 160/100 mm Hg. A single drug may be adequate in some patients with BPs less than 160/100 mm Hg. The presence of risk factors (such as diabetes, smoking, obesity, high blood cholesterol, or a family history of a heart attack or stroke at a relatively young age) or evidence of pathologic changes caused by hypertension (such as heart disease, stroke, kidney function impairment, or damage to the arteries of the eyes or legs) necessitates the use of a more-intensive treatment. Your physician will usually select a combination of drugs that most effectively treats your particular type of hypertension and risk factors.

In general, when lifestyle changes (for example, weight loss, limitation of salt and alcohol consumption, and increased exercise) do not normalize the BP, antihypertensive drugs should be started with the objective of lowering BP to a level of about 130/80 mm Hg or less. In the presence of diabetes or kidney failure, the BP goal should preferably be less than 130/80 mm Hg. In those individuals requiring antihypertensive medication, one drug adequately controls high BP in almost 50 percent of patients with stage 1 hypertension, up to 160/100 mm Hg. With stage 2 hypertension (a systolic BP equal to or greater than 160 mm Hg or a diastolic pressure equal to or greater than 100 mm Hg), two antihypertensive drugs will be sufficient to normalize BP in approximately 80 percent of hypertensives. Additional medication will be required for individuals who prove more resistant to treatment. The ways in which oral antihypertensive drugs work and their side effects were discussed in Question 66. Here we make some general comments about the use of these medications and then describe indications for specific drugs for patients with hypertension complicated by a variety of other medical conditions.

A long-acting thiazide diuretic (water pill) is often recommended as initial therapy in individuals with primary hypertension (that is, patients in whom all known causes of secondary hypertension have been eliminated) who have no significant impairment of kidney function and no history of gout (joint inflammation). Because diuretics can cause a loss of potassium in the urine, some doctors prefer to use a small-to-moderate dose of a potassium-sparing diuretic and periodically check the effect of this drug on the serum concentration of potassium. The rare occurrence of impotence in some men may require discontinuance.

Even small doses of thiazide diuretics will normalize BP in about 50 percent of individuals, and these agents are among the least expensive of all antihypertensive drugs. Diuretics are particularly effective in older adults (especially in patients with only systolic hypertension) and in African Americans and other individuals with salt-sensitive hypertension (that is, in individuals who retain salt).

Diuretics and beta blockers have the longest track record in treating hypertension, and their ability to decrease the disease complications associated with hypertension and mortality from hypertension has been established by many carefully controlled studies.

Beta blockers have been available for many years and are being used more often to treat hypertension. Most beta blockers lower BP by dilating arteries and reducing the rate and pumping force of the heart, which decreases BP. Beta blockers are not recommended for the initial treatment of patients with uncomplicated hypertension. They are contraindicated or should be used cautiously if the patient has a history of asthma or chronic lung disease that could be aggravated by the constriction of air passages in the lungs — an effect sometimes linked to these drugs. Furthermore, beta blockers should not be given to patients with any impairment of the electrical conduction system in the heart, as they could further slow the conduction system and the heart rate.

These drugs have been shown to be of value in the treatment of some forms of heart failure. Because they decrease the rate and pumping force of the normal heart and prevent these processes from increasing much during exercise, beta blockers are not recommended for athletes or patients who are very physically active. On the other hand, the decreased rate and work of the heart lessens its need for oxygen, which is beneficial for patients with angina (pain or pressure sensation in the chest caused by failure of oxygen reaching the heart). Therefore, beta blockers are a good choice for patients with angina or for those who have had a heart attack. Strong evidence also indicates that these drugs may reduce the risk of a second heart attack, which is a compelling reason for their use following a heart attack in individuals with or without hypertension.

Angiotensin-converting enzyme (ACE) inhibitors are as effective as diuretics and beta blockers at lowering BP. Except for a dry, hacking cough in 10 to 20 percent of patients, these agents produce few side effects and rarely cause impotence. As a result, they have become very popular antihypertensive medications. ACE inhibitors' ability to prevent or slow kidney damage in patients with diabetes, and their beneficial effects in patients with heart failure, especially if hypertension is present, or following a heart attack, have further increased their popularity. An ACE inhibitor may improve the antihypertensive effect of most antihypertensive medications, especially when used in combination with a diuretic.

Angiotensin receptor blockers (ARBs) are as effective as the ACE inhibitors and have the advantage of not causing a cough and very rarely causing a serious hypersensitivity reaction. They seem to match all of the beneficial effects of the ACE inhibitors.

Calcium-channel blockers have become very popular antihypertensive drugs. Only the long-acting drugs are currently recommended, because short-acting calcium-channel blockers can cause a drop in BP and an increase in heart rate. The ability of the long-acting versions to lower BP is similar to that of other antihypertensive medications. Calcium-channel blockers appear particularly effective in older people, African Americans, and sodium-sensitive individuals. Because the nondihydropyridine calcium-channel blockers decrease the electrical conduction in the heart, they should not be used in patients who take beta blockers and in patients who already have some slowing of conduction in the heart. Calcium-channel blockers may occasionally cause ankle edema, and, very rarely, swelling of the gums.

Alpha$_1$ blockers are typically used when a normalization of BP is not achieved with a combination of the other antihypertensive drugs. These agents improve urinary flow in some men who suffer urinary obstruction due to an enlarged prostate. In addition, they also may lower total cholesterol and triglycerides and increase "good" cholesterol (HDL), which may make them useful to some physically active individuals for whom beta blockers would be contraindicated.

Alpha$_2$ agonists [e.g., clonidine (Catapres)], which act mainly in the brain, are not usually chosen to treat hypertension because of their side effects of sedation and an annoying dry mouth sensation. However, alpha-methyldopa (Aldomet) is the antihypertensive drug most frequently used to treat hypertension during pregnancy, as it has been shown to be effective and safe for both mother and fetus.

> Treatment of hypertension should be tailored to suit each patient and to ensure maximum benefits, as the drugs prescribed for some individuals are determined by the history of a medical condition or a coexistent disease.

Many combinations of antihypertensive drugs have become available (see Question 66). Because of their convenience, combinations of two or even three antihypertensive drugs in one pill have increased in popularity. Of course it is impossible to determine how effective each drug is when it is given in combination or to determine whether only one of the drugs in proper dosage might be adequate to normalize mild (stage 1) hypertension. Given that at least two drugs will be required to normalize BP in at least 80 percent of patients with stage 2 hypertension, and even for many stage 1 hypertensives, starting treatment with a combination of drugs seems very reasonable. Furthermore, to lower BP, small doses of each drug in combination will result in fewer side effects than a large dose of a single medication.

Rarely, potent vasodilators are required in circumstances in which other medications are unable to normalize the BP. And some of the older drugs (in particular, adrenergic depleters) are rarely used today because of their potential side effects and because other drugs can better control hypertension.

In summary, treatment of hypertension should be tailored to suit each patient and to ensure maximum benefits, as the drugs prescribed for some individuals are determined by the history of a medical condition or a coexistent disease. Weight reduction for patients who are overweight or obese, limitation of salt and alcohol intake, and appropriate exercise are always indicated. Of extreme importance is quitting cigarette smoking, because smoking can accelerate damage to the blood vessels of the heart, brain, and elsewhere (see Question 51). In a smoker, the presence of hypertension further increases the chance of a heart attack and stroke and of obstruction of blood flow in the legs.

In general, treatment of an individual with stage 1 hypertension (less than 160/100 mm Hg) and without any history or current evidence of disease can initially consist of a long-acting thiazide diuretic (water pill). If the patient has any of the more severe complications of hypertension, a higher BP, or very severe malignant hypertension, then more intensive treatment — sometimes requiring intravenous drugs and even hospitalization — will be needed. An ACE inhibitor, an ARB, or a calcium-channel blocker may also be effective as the initiating treatment.

A good reason for initiating treatment with a diuretic is that this type of drug has been shown to reduce cardiovascular events and death. Perhaps 50 to 60 percent of hypertensives are salt sensitive. Diuretics are especially effective for these patients, because they eliminate salt and water retention. Diuretics can significantly enhance the effectiveness of other antihypertensive drugs — especially the ACE inhibitors and ARBs. Normalization of BP to levels below 130/80 mm Hg often requires a combination of two drugs, and occasionally a combination of three or four drugs.

It is impossible to predict with certainty who will respond best to a specific antihypertensive drug and who will or will not tolerate the drug, so selection of a specific antihypertensive medication and the appropriate dosage depends somewhat on trial and observation, and requires close cooperation between the doctor and patient. Certain medical conditions may preclude the use of some antihypertensive drugs, whereas some drugs are specifically indicated with coexisting medical conditions. Consult your physician to determine when certain drugs are indicated or contraindicated (see Table 9).

Table 9. Special Circumstances when Various Antihypertensive Drugs May Be Indicated or Contraindicated for the Treatment of Hypertension

Drug	Indications	Contraindications
Alpha₁ antagonists	• Men with urination difficulty because of prostate enlargement • May decrease "bad" cholesterol (LDL) and triglycerides and increase "good" cholesterol (HDL)	• Use with caution in patients prone to fainting
Alpha₂ agonists	• Pregnancy (only Aldomet) • Hypertension not controlled by other drugs • People experiencing panic attacks and symptoms resulting from withdrawal of addictive drugs	
Beta blockers	• Prevention of a second heart attack • Chest pain or pressure sensation (angina) due to poor blood supply to heart • Cases where the heart muscle is excessively thick, which impairs heart function • Heart failure • Some irregularities of heart rhythm • Some cases with rapid heart rate due to overactive thyroid gland • Some types of hand tremor • Migraine	• Impaired electrical conduction in heart (heart block) • Very slow heart rate • Asthma and lung disease with airway obstruction (e.g., chronic bronchitis or emphysema) • Athletes and young, physically very active people
Calcium-channel blockers	• Chest pain or pressure sensation (angina) due to poor blood supply to heart • Poor circulation in the legs • Some irregularities of heart rhythm (nondihydropyridines) • Older people and African Americans (especially with systolic hypertension) • Migraine (nondihydropyridines)	• Use with caution in patients receiving beta blockers, as some calcium-channel blockers (nondihydropyridines) may further impair electrical conduction in the heart

(cont'd.)

Table 9. Special Circumstances when Various Antihypertensive Drugs May Be Indicated or Contraindicated for the Treatment of Hypertension (cont'd.)

Drug	Indications	Contraindications
Combina-tion alpha$_1$ and beta blocker	• Heart failure, but only Coreg (carvediol) is recommended	
Direct vasodilators	• Cases where hypertension is very difficult to control (however, be-cause they cause a rapid heartbeat and water retention, a beta blocker and diuretic should be used in addi-tion to the direct vasodilator)	
Thiazide diuretic	• Heart failure • Salt-sensitive hypertension (es-pecially in African Americans) • Older people (especially with only systolic hypertension) • Osteoporosis	• History of gout (painful, inflamed joints) • Impairment of kid-ney function
Vasodilating beta block-ers, ACE in-hibitors, and angiotensin blockers	• Diabetes, especially with kidney damage • Heart failure • Following heart attack in some patients	• Pregnancy • Use with caution in patients with kidney disease, as may retain potassium

The ultimate goal of antihypertensive treatment is to prevent any negative complications related to hypertension by reducing BP to normal levels. With the drugs available today, BP can be controlled successfully in almost all patients who are motivated to work with their physician to determine the proper drug or combi-nation of drugs and dosages for successful treatment. Specialists in hypertension should be consulted regarding patients who are difficult to manage. It is a remarkable achievement that lifestyle changes and antihypertensive therapy have helped reduce the number of stroke and heart fatalities by 60 percent and 54 per-cent, respectively, in the past twenty-five years!

70 Should I Use Aspirin if I Have Hypertension?

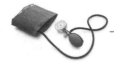

Patients with hypertension should first normalize their blood pressure. Then, if there are no contraindications (such as a history of an ulcer of the digestive tract, any bleeding tendency, sensitivity to aspirin or any of the nonsteroidal anti-inflammatory drugs [NSAIDs], or use of an anticoagulant such as Coumadin), patients are started on one baby aspirin daily (81 mg/day). Aspirin is especially indicated if the patient has a history of a heart attack, stroke, or transient ischemic attack (TIA, also known as a ministroke) and particularly in patients who are more than fifty years old.

> Patients with hypertension should first normalize their blood pressure. Then, if there are no contraindications, patients are started on one baby aspirin daily.

Aspirin is probably the most commonly used medication in most parts of the world. Its popularity derives from its ability to combat inflammation by blocking the effect of certain hormones called prostaglandins and to reduce or eliminate all sorts of pain, whether the pain is acute and temporary or even chronic, as occurs in arthritis. In addition, aspirin interferes with blood clotting by preventing platelets (very small cell-like structures in the blood) from sticking to one another, as they normally do, to help form blood clots when needed. This anticlotting effect likely explains why aspirin reduces the risk of a first heart attack, improves survival of patients who have had a heart attack, and reduces the chance of another heart attack by as much as 50 percent. Furthermore, this drug reduces the chance of a heart attack and death in patients with chest pain or pressure sensation (angina) due to poor circulation to the heart muscle. Evidence indicates that aspirin can reduce by 20 percent the occurrence of a stroke in individuals who have already had a nonhemorrhagic stroke or a TIA that resulted from a clot formation in a vessel supplying blood to the brain. Because some strokes result from a hemorrhage in the brain, aspirin should not be used if there is any evidence of such bleeding, as it might increase the bleeding.

Blood clots may form in vessels of the brain that become narrowed by atherosclerosis (hardening of the arteries due to excessive accumulation of cholesterol) or they may form elsewhere in the body (such as in the large arteries of the neck or in the heart) and may travel in the circulation and reach the brain, where they can block the circulation and cause brain damage. Aspirin may reduce the chances that such clots will form; however, to prevent clots in the heart produced by an irregular heartbeat (atrial fibrillation), another anticlotting agent, warfarin (Coumadin), has proven to be more effective than aspirin.

Aspirin may irritate the lining of the stomach and intestinal tract and cause some bleeding. It may also aggravate or cause ulceration, sometimes causing severe bleeding. Therefore, patients with ulcers or those who develop abdominal complaints such as pain or "indigestion" should not use aspirin or nonsteroidal anti-inflammatory drugs (NSAIDs) such as Advil, Motrin, Nuprin, Naprosyn, Indocin, Clinoril, Ansaid, or Aleve. Smaller doses of aspirin, such as a baby aspirin (81 mg/day), may be just as effective as — or even more effective than — a regular aspirin (325 mg/day) in preventing heart attacks and strokes due to blood clots. A possible explanation for this phenomenon is that lower doses of aspirin can block the ag-

> Patients with ulcers or those who develop abdominal complaints such as pain or "indigestion" should not use aspirin or nonsteroidal anti-inflammatory drugs (NSAIDs).

gregation (sticking together) of platelets by thromboxane, a hormone that makes platelets more sticky and causes blood vessels to constrict. Both effects (prevention of platelet aggregation and blood vessel constriction) are undesirable, because they would promote the formation of a clot. On the other hand, a low dose of aspirin (unlike a high dose) does not inhibit formation of prostacyclin, a hormone that prevents platelet stickiness, promotes the dilation of blood vessels, and thereby prevents clot formation. If intestinal bleeding is caused by aspirin, the use of aspirin should be discontinued immediately until the bleeding has stopped. However, some believe that in patients who have had a stroke or heart attack, aspirin use should be restarted because of its effectiveness in preventing a recurrence of these conditions. The addition of an antacid (e.g., an H2 antagonist or a PPI, i.e., a protein pump inhibitor) may be used to reduce the possibility of recurrent bleeding.

NSAIDs, when taken repeatedly and especially for prolonged periods, may reduce the effectiveness of diuretics (water pills) because their effect on the kidneys can cause salt and water retention. Furthermore, they can decrease the production of hormones that dilate blood vessels and reduce the effectiveness of various drugs used to lower blood pressure. When taken only occasionally, NSAIDs do not interfere with blood pressure control. *Aspirin does not seem to interfere significantly with blood pressure control of hypertensive patients, unlike most other NSAIDs, when used repeatedly in large amounts.*

71 What Are Alternative Medicine and Herbal Medicine? Are They Helpful in Hypertension?

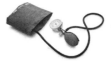

The term alternative medicine is here used mainly to describe a number of therapeutic procedures that are not generally employed by medical doctors to treat disease. On the other hand, the use of herbal remedies combined with healthy food has also been designated "alternative medicine" and may sometimes be helpful in treating certain medical conditions.

Alternative medicine and herbal medicine have been developing a large following as many Americans become more health conscious. However, while evidence of their clear benefit is being collected, some of the public may be misled by unsubstantiated claims about the benefits of alternative treatments. These claims made in newspapers and magazines, or on television, radio, or the Internet, and the vigorous endorsement of alternative medical approaches on talk shows and by friends and acquaintances can convince many Americans to use untested treatments and procedures, many of which are very expensive and some of which can be harmful.

These procedures include, among others, chelation therapy, homeopathy, acupuncture, chiropractic treatment, massage, biofeedback, meditation, and the use of various herbs and nutritional supplements. In recent years, an estimated 42 percent of Americans have used these unconventional treatments at a cost of more than $40 billion, most of which took the form of out-of-pocket expenses. Hypertension is among the top ten conditions for which individuals used alternative therapy, without consulting their physician, but there is as yet no convincing evidence that alternative medicine can control hypertension.

> There is as yet no convincing evidence that alternative medicine can control hypertension.

Chelation, for example, makes use of a chemical named EDTA (ethylenediaminetetraacetic acid), which is given intravenously to cleanse the blood. This technique can be an effective form of treatment for lead poisoning. However, claims that it can reduce hardening of the arteries and BP; normalize weight; lessen arthritis; reverse impotence, hair loss, and Alzheimer's disease; prevent chronic fatigue; reduce cancer mortality by 90 percent; and produce a youthful appearance are unproven. Moreover, chelation can lower calcium in the blood, resulting in serious irregularities of the heart, and cause respiratory arrest, muscle spasms, and kidney damage. Indeed, some patients have died as a result of chelation therapy.

Homeopathy is a therapeutic approach to treating disease that was originally developed by Dr. Samuel Hahnemann (1755–1843). He proposed that drugs that in ordinary amounts produce symptoms and signs or manifestations of a disease in healthy subjects should be used in very small amounts to treat patients with that disease. Although some physicians endorse this approach, it seems to us very unlikely that the extremely small doses of drugs used in homeopathy would have any significant effect on the disease process because it is recognized that the effectiveness of most drugs depends on adequate dosage. Much anecdotal evidence has been published to validate homeopathic therapy, but there is little scientific support for its efficacy in treating any disease, including hypertension.

Acupuncture does have some beneficial therapeutic applications, and many millions of acupuncture treatments are performed each year in the United States, particularly for the treatment of pain and addiction. Treatment includes inserting thin needles in certain areas of the body, which, practitioners claim, may stimulate nerves that send impulses to the spinal cord and brain and suppress pain pathways. It is noteworthy that in China acupuncture is sometimes used in place of anesthesia for surgical procedures. Pain severity is a subjective, difficult-to-measure sensation, thus complicating how to best evaluate acupuncture's effectiveness. In some cases, improvement may occur, but it is difficult to determine whether a patient's high expectation of improvement may have contributed to the benefit of acupuncture. Although some claim that acupuncture can lower high BP and raise low BP, no good evidence supports these claims.

Chiropractic treatments concentrate mainly on manipulations of the spine in an attempt to correct any misalignment of vertebrae, thereby relieving pressure on nerves and restoring normal nerve conduction to muscles and various organs of the body. Relief of some types of pain may occur, but claims that spinal manipulation is beneficial for a variety of diseases (unrelated to the spine or muscles) and that it can lower BP are unproven.

Another very popular form of alternative medicine involves a large variety of healthy food supplements and herbal remedies.

Some very important drugs were initially discovered in natural sources—for example, aspirin was found in willow tree bark; digitalis was present in the foxglove plant; a blood thinner was found in clover; and reserpine, a blood-pressure-lowering drug, was isolated from a root found in India. Garlic, when consumed in large amounts, may lower "bad" cholesterol and raise "good" cholesterol (see Questions 50 and 73); although a few reports claim that it may lower BP when taken in large amounts, most studies indicate that it has no such effect. Some herbs, such as licorice, have been shown to raise blood pressure. Virtually none of the commonly used herbs that can be obtained in health-food stores have been scientifically evaluated to determine their action, potency, and safety.

Though very widely available, herbal remedies can cause many harmful side effects, including death and serious interaction with prescription drugs (see Question 73). One should be aware of the hazards of these supplements and herbal remedies and consult a physician before using them (see Table 10 on page 152).

Finally, we should mention copper bracelets and magnets, which are purported to relieve all sorts of pain. Many people swear this simple "alternative" remedy brings them enormous benefits or can even cure a chronic pain. Magnets are usually placed in the bed under the mattress and, following one night's sleep, miraculous cures of backaches have been reported. Unfortunately, no scientific studies have documented these anecdotal reports—that is, no studies have compared the beneficial effects of magnets with similar-appearing objects that have no magnetic properties. This form of alternative medicine has no place in the treatment of hypertension, and it is important that patients with heart pacemakers avoid close contact with strong magnets.

The benefits of alternative medicine may sometimes be related to the "placebo effect." A placebo (the word derives from Latin meaning "I will please") is defined as a "dummy medical treatment": a medicinal preparation or treatment that has no specific known pharmacologic activity against the patient's illness or complaint (see Question 74). The beneficial effects of placebos are best explained by the psychophysiological effects experienced by the patient who has high expectations for improvement.

In conclusion, if you are considering alternative medicine, we strongly urge you to be cautious and consult your physician before using any such remedies. More important, leaving your BP untreated or inadequately treated, especially when there are lifestyle changes that can be beneficial, such as following the DASH diet, reducing salt consumption, increasing physical activity, losing weight, and reducing alcohol consumption as well as the use of safe and well-tolerated drugs that have been proven to lower BP and prevent heart attacks, strokes, renal disease, and heart failure, are a far better way to manage high BP.

72 Are Relaxation and Biofeedback Techniques Effective in Hypertension Management?

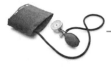

Some members of the public continue to believe that relaxation and biofeedback techniques can be of therapeutic value in the management of primary hypertension, the most common form of hypertension, for which the cause remains unknown. While these techniques may lower blood pressure (BP) for a short time, no studies have demonstrated that they can keep BP lowered for a prolonged period of time.

A number of relaxation procedures may improve a person's sense of well-being and relieve tension and nervousness. In essence, these techniques are a form of stress management, and they depend, to a major extent, on the relaxation of major muscles of the body. In addition, hypnosis, Zen meditation, yoga, and transcendental meditation require mental concentration ("to clear the mind of all distractions") and sometimes the repetition of a word or sound by the individual. Relaxation may be so pronounced that brain wave studies (electroencephalogram changes) indicate a pattern similar to that seen during sleep. As a result of this profound degree of relaxation, the activity of the nervous system diminishes. A decrease in sympathetic nerve activity is accompanied by a slowing of the heart rate and a dilation of arteries, which results in a modest degree of BP reduction. This reduction is only temporary, however.

Biofeedback is designed to help an individual sense or feel a change in a bodily function, such as heart rate and BP. With instruments that can convey information about BP, heart rate, or the degree of muscle contraction to the individual participating in biofeedback, systolic and diastolic pressures may be temporarily reduced by as much as 20 and 10 mm Hg.

It is very apparent that stress results in an elevation of BP, whereas mental and muscular relaxation are accompanied by a decrease in BP. For example, most individuals' BP is at least 5 mm Hg higher while at work than that it is when they are more relaxed at home in the evening.

The lowering of BP achievable with relaxation techniques and biofeedback is usually only temporary. After terminating one or a series of these procedures, BP returns to the level present before the relaxation or biofeedback procedures began. It must be concluded that these techniques, although of interest experimentally, may not have therapeutic value in the long-term management of hypertension. However, a recently developed and approved instrument called RespeRate has utilized these techniques and shows long-term BP reductions. The device guides patients, by tones they hear from headphones, to increase inspiration and slow expiration to less than ten breaths per minute. If the device is used for fifteen minutes daily at least three times each week, it appears effective in significantly reducing elevated BP by dilating blood vessels. A number of studies have established that this device may be helpful in preventing and controlling hypertension, whether or not patients are taking antihypertensive drugs.

73 Are Health-Food Supplements, Herbal Remedies, and "Body Builders" Good for You? Can They Affect Your Blood Pressure, and Can They Be Harmful?

A very strong interest in the value of health-food supplements and herbal remedies has developed throughout the United States in the past few decades, and the demand for them continues to increase dramatically. To date, no regulation of the quality and strength of herbal remedies has been established. As already mentioned, while some herbs have been helpful in treating hypertension, others may be harmful and even cause serious interactions with prescription drugs.

Table 10 lists some popular health-food supplements and herbal remedies and their side effects, as reported by the Mayo Clinic. For instance, a variety of "natural" diuretics have been advocated to increase the elimination of salt and water, even though no evidence shows that they are efficacious in lowering blood pressure. In addition, soy protein in large amounts may decrease "bad" cholesterol but has no effect on blood pressure.

Table 10. Selected Food Supplements and Their Purported Health Claims

Food Supplements Promoted as Lowering Blood Pressure	
Supplement	Comments/Potential Side Effects
Coenzyme Q-10	No good evidence that it lowers blood pressure
Garlic	Large doses can lower "bad" cholesterol without changing "good" cholesterol. Garlic does not lower blood pressure.
Ginkgo biloba	No good evidence that it lowers blood pressure
Green tea	No good evidence that it lowers blood pressure
Omega-3 polyunsaturated fatty acids (in fish oil)	Large doses may lower blood pressure (and triglycerides) and can reduce blood clotting, but they have little if any effect on cholesterol

(cont'd.)

Table 10. Selected Food Supplements and Their Purported Health Claims (cont'd.)

Supplement	Comments/Potential Side Effects
Vitamin C	No good evidence that it lowers blood pressure
Supplements Promoted as Increasing Blood Pressure	
Supplement	Comments/Potential Side Effects
Ephedrine (ephedra)	Can cause a dangerous rise in blood pressure
Licorice root	Can increase blood pressure
Yohimbine	Can increase blood pressure
Herbal Remedies	
Supplement	Comments/Potential Side Effects
Aloe	Increased toxicity of some drugs used to treat heart failure; abdominal cramps
Aristolochia fangchi	Kidney failure, cancer of the urinary tract
Comfrey	Liver failure
Echinacea	Suppression of the immune system
Feverfew	Interaction with anticoagulants to increase bleeding
Ginkgo biloba	Bleeding in eye if given with aspirin, bleeding in the brain, inhibition of blood clotting
Ginseng	Nervousness, excitement, headache, insomnia, and palpitations. May elevate blood pressure. May cause falsely elevated digoxin blood levels and mislead physician to pursue an inappropriate treatment.
Kava-kava	Muscle weakness, skin discoloration
Ma huang	Stroke, heart attack, rapid heart rate, and sudden death
Saw palmetto	Diarrhea, upset stomach
St. John's wort	May augment depression, if the user is taking an antidepressant; sun sensitivity; interactions with blood pressure drugs. Can decrease the effectiveness of medications for AIDS and heart transplants.
Valerian	Sedative effect causing drowsiness

After many occurrences of serious side effects, ephedra has finally been restricted. The fact that ephedra's main ingredient is ephedrine makes this herbal "remedy" a potentially very dangerous substance. Like amphetamines, it can stimulate the nervous system and produce side effects including hypertension, a rapid heart rate, anxiety, insomnia, psychosis, heart attack, stroke, and death.

> Ephedra's main ingredient—ephedrine—renders this herbal "remedy" a potentially very dangerous substance. Like amphetamines, it can stimulate the nervous system and produce side effects including hypertension, a rapid heart rate, anxiety, insomnia, psychosis, heart attack, stroke, and death.

Although many over-the-counter drugs contain ephedrine, the concentration of ephedrine is indicated on the packaging and these drugs are regulated by the Food and Drug Administration, so the Food and Drug Administration's guidance on the use of these drugs is always available. In contrast, the concentration of ephedrine in ephedra preparations may vary considerably and certainly may be dangerous to consume, especially in large amounts.

The use of "body builders" such as anabolic steroids or gamma-hydroxybutyrate (GHB) may cause severe illness, and occasionally death. Steroids may cause the retention of salt and water, which can elevate blood pressure. Furthermore, they may markedly decrease HDL (high density lipoprotein, the "good" cholesterol). The use of body builders is not recommended.

No one should risk using herbal products about which they know little or nothing. Some herbal products are often spiked with drugs and contaminants not listed on the labels that could be harmful. Check with your doctor before using herbal remedies and health-food supplements if you don't know whether they contain contaminants that could be harmful.

74. What Is the Placebo Effect?

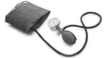

A placebo is defined as "an inert, inactive, innocuous, harmless substance, or a dummy medical treatment, that has no effect on bodily functions." It is used as a control when evaluating the therapeutic effectiveness of a drug or procedure (see Questions 7 and 71). The word *placebo* actually means "I shall please" (in Latin). Often an inert substance with no pharmacologically active ingredients (such as a sugar or starch pill) when ingested, a placebo can appear to exert various beneficial effects — a phenomenon known as the placebo effect. Therefore, to establish the benefit of a drug or procedure, the therapeutic efficacy of the proposed treatment must be significantly greater than that of a placebo.

> Often an inert substance with no pharmacologically active ingredients, when ingested, can appear to exert various beneficial effects—a phenomenon known as the placebo effect.

In clinical studies, it is important that neither the patient nor the doctor administering a drug or placebo knows which is the drug and which is the placebo. Such a double-blind study eliminates any bias from the patient or doctor in analyzing and assessing the effects of a drug.

Placebos have been shown to reduce systolic blood pressure by 5 to 10 mm Hg and diastolic blood pressure by 3 to 5 mm Hg; they can also cause "side effects" such as headache, sexual dysfunction, weakness, fatigue, and dizziness. In some comparative trials, the placebo caused just as many side effects as the active drug and, in some instances, caused even more side effects! How can this happen?

Expectations about and anticipation of a benefit from any substance or procedure can result in a significant placebo effect, that is, an improvement — regardless of whether the drug or procedure has any real therapeutic value. The warmth and caring shown by a sympathetic doctor can create a patient–physician relationship that raises the patient's hope and improves their mood and well-being. The improved mood change can contribute to the placebo effect. Even an abnormal objective finding, such as elevated blood pressure, may improve with the use of some innocuous but awesome-looking machine that impresses the patient by harmlessly emitting sounds and lights, which the patient believes are therapeutic. Repeated treatments with such a dramatically impressive device were reported by the late Dr. William Goldring, an authority on hypertension, and his colleagues at New York University Medical Center to cause a pronounced lowering of blood pressure related directly to the placebo effect. Hypertension invariably returned to pretreatment levels after treatment was discontinued, however. This placebo effect most likely resulted from reduced emotional stress and probably a decreased activity of the sympathetic nervous system, which resulted in dilation of the arteries and a reduction in blood pressure. According to Dr. Herbert Spiegel, the placebo effect can occur "when conditions are optimal for hope, faith, trust, and love."

The power of suggestion from friends and acquaintances that a certain procedure or herbal remedy may relieve a variety of symptoms or conditions may have dramatic effects. Infinite anecdotal claims and testimonials have been made about alternative forms of treatment (see Question 71), suggesting that such remedies can result in miraculous cures of even long-standing medical problems. For example, claims have been made that chronic backaches may sometimes be cured by sleeping on a bed with magnets placed beneath the mattress. Those claiming cures of their backaches are absolutely convinced that the magnets were responsible for the cure. Although this explanation seems highly unlikely, we can test this theory by placing magnets under the mattresses of one series of beds and nonmagnetized objects, which appear identical to the magnets, under the mattresses of another series of beds. Individuals with backaches can then report any benefit from sleeping in these beds. If essentially no significant difference is seen in backache improvement between those sleeping over magnets versus those sleeping in beds with nonmagnetized objects, then any improvement must be attributed to a placebo effect. No such trial has ever been conducted.

The importance of understanding and recognizing the placebo effect cannot be overstated. In the final analysis, one must appreciate the significance of the placebo effect before accepting any unproved form of treatment as being responsible for a therapeutic effect. The public should be alerted to recognize that benefits from various types of alternative medicine, herbal remedies, and "health" foods (see Questions 71 and 73) may result from a placebo effect, rather than from any realistic medicinal action. One must also remember that the use of some alternative medicines, herbs, and health foods can actually be harmful.

75 Are Vitamins Helpful in Treating People with Hypertension and Hypercholesterolemia? Can They Be Harmful?

The interest of the public in vitamins has increased enormously in recent years, reflecting the strong belief that some vitamins are valuable in treating a variety of diseases. Although the claims of health benefits may be overzealous, very compelling evidence does show that people who consume large amounts of fruits and vegetables have less cancer and heart disease. Some also claim, but have not yet proved, that vitamin C (ascorbic acid) and vitamin E (alphatocopherol) — both of which are antioxidants — may prevent arterial damage and the deleterious effects of harmful oxidation products known as superoxides (see Question 96). Therefore, it seems reasonable to eat more fruits and vegetables as part of a healthy diet. It is well known that consumption of increased amounts of vitamin D is important for healthy bones; however, recent evidence also suggests that large doses of vitamin D may be of value in preventing heart disease and stroke.

Vitamin E has no effect on blood pressure or blood lipids (cholesterol and triglycerides), even when consumed in large amounts. Vitamin C may lower blood cholesterol, but this change is relatively minor, and daily supplements of 500 mg appear necessary for this effect. Therefore, there is no reason to take large amounts of vitamin C to lower cholesterol.

> *Vitamin C (ascorbic acid) and vitamin E (alphatocopherol)— both antioxidants— may prevent arterial damage and the deleterious effects of harmful oxidation products known as superoxides. Vitamin E has no effect on blood pressure or blood lipids, whereas vitamin C may lower blood cholesterol to a minor extent.*

Although there has been much talk about the ability of large amounts (megadoses) of vitamin C to prevent the common cold, this claim has been scientifically investigated and never substantiated. Furthermore, it has been reported that megadoses of more than 1,000 mg can cause kidney stones, increase blood levels of estrogen in women taking estrogen, interfere with the absorption of vitamin B-12, and cause scurvy in the offspring of some mothers on megadoses.

Niacin (vitamin B-3, nicotinic acid) can effectively lower "bad" cholesterol (LDL—low-density lipoprotein), elevate "good" cholesterol (HDL—high-density lipoprotein), and reduce triglycerides. All these lipid (fat) changes can help prevent or minimize atherosclerosis (damaging of the lining of arteries), thereby reducing and possibly reversing any impairment of blood flow to vital organs. As with other drugs that lower LDL cholesterol, mortality from heart attacks may be reduced. *Niacin does not, however, lower blood pressure.* Unfortunately, its use to treat lipid abnormalities is frequently accompanied by a number of side effects, such as flushing, itching, intestinal upsets, stomach ulcers, gout (due to increased uric acid), difficulty controlling blood sugar (in diabetics, because niacin increases blood sugar), aggravation of asthma, and impairment of liver function, sometimes with jaundice. Rarely, a pronounced transitory decrease in blood pressure may occur. A combination of aspirin with niacin can reduce flushing and itching, which are the most common and annoying side effects. There are many other drugs available that can effectively treat abnormalities of blood fats with few side effects. Folic acid is valuable in preventing atherosclerosis, apparently working by preventing elevated blood levels of homocysteine (an amino acid — a substance that builds protein). Since it has been estimated that 40 percent of the U.S. population consumes inadequate amounts of folic acid, it would seem prudent for Americans to consume more folic acid. Folic acid does not have any effect on blood pressure, cholesterol, or triglycerides.

Other vitamins do not appear to have any effect in treating hypertension or hypercholesterolemia. It is noteworthy, however, that toxic doses of vitamin D may significantly increase calcium in the blood, which might then cause hypertension.

76 Will Hypertension or Antihypertensive Drugs Affect My Sex Life, and What about Use of Viagra or Special Food Supplements to Enhance Sexual Function?

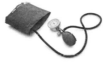

Hypertension alone (without the presence of any negative complications) may affect your sex life, causing impaired sexual function that sometimes improves after blood pressure is reduced with antihypertensive drugs. Nevertheless, impotence (inability to obtain or maintain an erection, impaired erectile function) or a lack of desire for sex (libido) is often psychogenic in origin (that is, due to mental and emotional attitude). Impaired blood supply to the penis due to obstruction by atherosclerosis of the arteries in the penis, sometimes the result of hypertension, can cause impotence — especially in older men. Failure to adequately perform sexual intercourse can cause considerable anxiety and depression in men and can cause disappointment and even anger in the spouse, which can lead to a disturbed relationship.

Sexual dysfunction has mainly been reported to affect many normotensive men between the ages of forty and seventy. It is conceivable that this rate of dysfunction might be even greater in hypertensive males on no medications, as concern over the presence of hypertension could cause additional anxiety and further compound the problem. As noted above, impotence may be caused by psychogenic problems, although atherosclerosis with impairment of blood flow to the penis is also a common cause. In addition, conditions that damage the nerves that control the erectile function of the penis (such as diabetes), as well as a deficiency of the male hormone testosterone, may lead to sexual dysfunction. Abnormal blood flow problems in the penis can be accurately identified by Doppler ultrasonography, and a deficiency of testosterone can be determined by a blood test.

Most antihypertensive drugs rarely cause impotence. Some beta blockers (e.g., propranolol) may occasionally be responsible for sexual dysfunction in men. Originally, diuretics were thought to cause impotence in some hypertensive men; however, recent evidence indicates these drugs do not cause sexual dysfunction. No remarkable change in sexual performance was experienced in men or women taking alpha$_1$ blockers, ACE inhibitors, or calcium-channel blockers. Angiotensin receptor blockers (ARBs) may even have a beneficial effect on impotence. (Some of the older sympathetic-nerve-blocking drugs may interfere with sexual function, but they are very rarely used or are not available to treat hypertension today.) Spironolactone is rarely used to treat primary hypertension, but it has been found to help some patients with congestive heart failure; since it can cause enlargement of the breasts in men and loss of sexual desire, a more recent and similar acting medication, eplerenone, may be preferable in men because it does not cause these undesirable side effects. In the event that the patient believes an antihypertensive drug has decreased their sexual function, the drug may be discontinued by the physician, if necessary, and another drug used. In most cases, however, the antihypertensive medication will probably not be the root cause of the impotence. In fact, in one large clinical trial the reported rate of impotency was greater in the placebo group than in the treated hypertensive group who, by the way, reported improved sexual response.

Sexual dysfunction has not been as well studied in women as it has been in men. Some women experienced a decrease in libido and/or lack of orgasmic response during intercourse after taking some of the drugs that were used to lower blood pressure in the past. None of the currently used medications to treat hypertension appear to cause sexual dysfunction in women, however.

Viagra, Cialis, and Levitra dilate blood vessels and improve blood flow to the penis by enhancing the effect of nitric oxide. These drugs can be used in patients with hypertension that is adequately controlled with medication or

Most antihypertensive drugs probably do not cause impotence. Diuretics and beta blockers may rarely be responsible for sexual dysfunction in men, but no remarkable change in sexual performance was experienced in men or women taking alpha$_1$ blockers, ACE inhibitors, or calcium-channel blockers.

lifestyle changes. Their use may be contraindicated in some patients with coronary heart disease, especially those who have angina, a history of recent heart attack, or congestive heart failure, or those who are also taking nitrates that may cause a pronounced drop in blood pressure. However, these drugs should not be prescribed to patients taking nitrates (those used to dilate arteries, e.g., nitroglycerine, Nitro-Bid, Nitrostat, Nitrol, Nitro-Dur, Isordil, Sorbitrate, Dilatrate, Imdur, Ismo, Cardilate, and others), as this combination may cause a dangerous decrease in blood pressure. If these drugs prove ineffective in restoring sexual function, a physician specializing in this type of disorder should be consulted. Sexual function can usually be restored.

No scientific evidence has shown that any food supplements are helpful in restoring sexual dysfunction.

77 Is There Any Danger That My Blood Pressure May Be Reduced Too Much with Medication?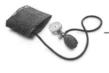

It is unlikely that antihypertensive medications will lead to too-low blood pressure (BP). Indeed, it is much more likely that your BP will not be reduced enough to protect you fully from the bad consequences of high BP. A recent survey indicated that only 37 percent of hypertensives in the United States had their BP controlled to 140/90 mm Hg or less.

Some older medications, most of which are not prescribed today, had a greater effect on the BP in the standing position than in the sitting or reclining position. They therefore produced light-headedness or even fainting when patients stood up rapidly. Most currently prescribed medications do not reduce the BP excessively in the standing position. However, such postural hypotension may occur in people over age sixty-five or in diabetic people and could be increased in those people given potent antihypertensive drugs. If symptoms such as dizziness occur when first standing, the physician will measure the BP in both the standing and sitting (or reclining) positions, before and after the patient has started medication to determine whether any excessive lowering of the BP occurs on standing.

78 Is There Any Danger in Changing My Antihypertensive Medication?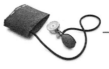

Changing your antihypertensive medication should not create problems if the change is made under the supervision of your physician. Many times, if your blood pressure (BP) is not well controlled, adding or substituting BP medications will bring the BP down. You should never stop a medication entirely without consulting your doctor (see Question 66). Abrupt cessation of a beta blocker in a patient with coronary artery disease, for example, may sometimes aggravate chest pain or pressure sensation (angina) or even cause a heart attack. Suddenly discontinuing a relatively high dose of clonidine (Catapres) may occasionally cause a significant elevation of BP.

If undesirable side effects are the reason for changing medication, be sure to discuss the problem with your doctor. Sometimes, using multiple medications in small doses will reduce or eliminate side effects and control the BP more effectively than using larger doses of single agents.

79 Why Is Hypertension Sometimes Resistant to Treatment?

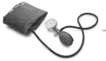

Hypertension is considered "resistant" to treatment when you still have a blood pressure above 140/90 mm Hg while taking at least three drugs in appropriate doses, all from different classes, one of which is a diuretic (see Table 8 on page 125). Generally, when high blood pressure does not respond to a good combination of drugs, patients are not taking the medications as prescribed. Eating too much salt, drinking too much alcohol, or taking large amounts of a non steroidal anti-inflammatory drug (NSAID) such as ibuprofen may also make high blood pressure less responsive to treatment. Obese patients are

Hypertension is not considered "resistant" to treatment until you have taken at least three drugs, all from different classes, including a diuretic.

more likely to be resistant to treatment than are thin patients, although the culprit may actually be falsely high readings taken in the obese arm.

When blood pressure remains high despite a good combination of drugs, one should suspect that some identifiable secondary form of hypertension is present. In these cases, the problem may follow from disease in a kidney artery, blocking the flow of blood to the kidney, a tumor of the adrenal gland (pheochromocytoma or aldosteronoma), or advanced kidney disease with kidney failure (see Question 38).

80 Can Hypertension Cause Pain in My Legs When I Walk?

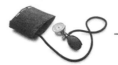

Hypertension can cause leg pain if it is associated with significant damage to the arteries supplying blood to the legs. Pain, ache, or fatigue that occurs in the legs, especially in the calf muscles, on walking and then subsides with rest is usually caused by impaired blood supply to the lower extremities. This type of pain, which is called intermittent claudication, results from atherosclerotic changes (that is, hardening of the arteries with obstruction of blood flow). Impairment of blood flow may also sometimes occur above the legs and cause pain in the hip, buttock, and thigh muscles on walking. If obstruction of blood flow is very severe, the patient may experience pain in the affected legs or feet, even when at rest. Surgical procedures may be able to improve blood supply to the legs, or in some cases a balloon attached to a catheter is used to open the obstruction. Occasionally, amputation of a foot or leg may be necessary with severely impaired blood supply and the development of gangrene. This latter negative complication occurs most commonly in diabetic patients and cigarette smokers. Therefore, early treatment to improve the blood supply is essential to prevent these types of complications.

In addition to hypertension, risk factors for the development of atherosclerosis include cigarette smoking, high levels of "bad" cholesterol (LDL — low-density lipoprotein) and low levels of "good" cholesterol (HDL — high-density lipoprotein), and diabetes mellitus. All of these risk factors can markedly enhance the occurrence of intermittent claudication, coronary disease (atherosclerosis of the coronary arteries in the heart), cerebrovascular disease (atherosclerosis of the arteries of the brain), and atherosclerotic changes in other important arteries, such as the carotid arteries of the neck (which supply blood to the brain) and the aorta (the largest artery, which carries blood away from the heart to all parts of the body). In general, the severity of the risk factors and their number are strongly correlated with the degree of atherosclerosis and its complications. Furthermore, because all of these negative complications tend to occur with aging, it is extremely important to control modifiable risk factors as soon as they are recognized. Quitting smoking is imperative (see Questions 51 and 52). In addition, every effort should be made to normalize an elevated blood pressure and LDL through lifestyle changes and medication, if necessary, and to control diabetes.

Leg pains (cramps) during exercise may result from a decreased level of potassium in the body. This condition can be easily identified by measuring the concentration of potassium in the blood. Leg cramps may also occur without exercise, especially at night. The cause of these leg cramps is not clear, and there is no consistently effective treatment for them. None of these cramps are related to primary hypertension.

81 What Is a Heart Attack?

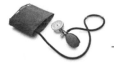

The term "heart attack" typically means a myocardial infarction, although it is sometimes used to describe impending infarction or spells of rapid or irregular heartbeats. *Infarction* means a death of some of the heart muscle, usually due to blockage of a coronary artery supplying blood to that area of muscle. Myocardial infarction can often be prevented by appropriate treatment of hypertension, high cholesterol, diabetes, and other risk factors, especially avoidance of cigarette smoking. Even in patients who have already had a heart attack, it is possible to prolong life and prevent recurrent heart attacks by appropriately treating high blood pressure, usually with a beta blocker, an ACE inhibitor, or both.

A heart attack is, of course, an acute emergency that your physician will want to treat as soon as possible. You should immediately report to your physician any pain or sensation of pressure or tightness in the chest that persists for more than a few minutes, particularly if the pain is very severe and extends into the back and neck or down the arms; it may be accompanied by sweating, nausea, and sometimes vomiting. Take one regular aspirin (unless you are allergic to aspirin) and go immediately to the nearest emergency room accompanied by a relative or friend, if possible. Angina (chest pain, a sensation of pressure, or tightness, sometimes with an extension of the pain into the jaw or down the left arm) is also caused by impaired blood supply to the heart. With angina, there is no death of heart muscle, however, and the symptoms are generally less severe, usually lasting for fewer than twenty minutes, and can be relieved by the application of nitroglycerin tablets, which dilate the arteries in the heart.

82 What Is Congestive Heart Failure? How Can It Be Prevented, and How Should It Be Treated?

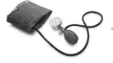

Heart failure occurs when the heart cannot pump blood effectively to the tissues of the body. When the pumping force becomes significantly impaired, blood backs up in the lungs, causing congestive heart failure. A number of conditions may cause congestive heart failure, including the following:

- hypertension
- damage of heart valves due to infection
- destruction of heart muscle caused by impaired blood supply, often as a result of a heart attack due to atherosclerosis and a blood clot in one of the coronary (heart) arteries
- destruction of heart muscle due to infections, excess alcohol consumption, and other causes

- congenital (inherited) abnormalities of the heart, its valves, or its blood vessels

Hypertension is present in an estimated 91 percent of patients who develop congestive heart failure. Indeed, hypertension is the major preventable factor in this very serious condition that claims 400,000 lives annually. Frequently the muscle fibers of the left ventricle (the muscular pumping chamber of the heart) become enlarged in response to the increased work required to maintain an adequate blood flow against an elevated blood pressure; this enlargement of the heart muscle is known as left ventricular hypertrophy (LVH; see Question 83). Similarly, hypertrophy (increased size) of skeletal muscles in the biceps of the arms or elsewhere occurs with repeated demand for increased muscular work, such as weightlifting exercise. If hypertension is left untreated, in which case it often worsens, the heart muscle becomes incapable of carrying out the excess work required to effectively pump blood to the tissues. At this point, congestive heart failure develops.

> *Heart failure occurs when the heart cannot pump blood effectively to the tissues of the body. When the pumping force becomes significantly impaired, blood backs up in the lungs, causing congestive heart failure.*

Adequate treatment of hypertension can markedly reduce mortality from stroke, heart attack, and congestive heart failure. Sadly, only 37 percent of the hypertensive population has their blood pressure under proper control. This poor success rate reflects the fact that many hypertensives are either unaware that they have hypertension or are receiving inadequate antihypertensive medication. The incidence of congestive heart failure is increasing in the United States partly because of the aging population, as older people are more apt to have hypertension and atherosclerosis. This disease is the most common hospital discharge diagnosis for Medicare patients (patients sixty-five years old or older).

Every effort should be made to detect hypertension as early as possible so that it can be managed appropriately. In addition, quitting smoking, controlling weight and cholesterol, and getting adequate exercise can help prevent the development of atherosclerosis and heart disease. Congestive heart failure is an ominous manifestation that requires hospitalization and usually treatment with ACE inhibitors or angiotensin receptor blockers (drugs that help prevent the deleterious effects of angiotensin), diuretics including spironolactone (Aldactone), salt limitation, digitalis, and sometimes additional drugs to control serious heart irregularities. Reducing risk factors — smoking, diabetes, hypertension, excess weight, elevated LDL (low-density lipoprotein, i.e., "bad" cholesterol) and triglycerides, a sedentary lifestyle, and excess sodium in the diet — is key to preventing or reducing the occurrence of congestive heart failure.

83 What Is Left Ventricular Hypertrophy?

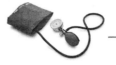

Left ventricular hypertrophy (LVH) is an enlargement of the muscle of the left ventricle, which is the main pumping chamber of the heart. If the heart must continuously work against increased pressure, it will, like any muscle, eventually enlarge due to overwork. The traditional analogy is the muscle in the blacksmith's arm, which, because of repeated pounding on the anvil, undergoes hypertrophy and becomes enlarged.

The best way of identifying LVH is to use an echocardiogram, which can visualize the size and configuration of the heart and the thickness of its muscular walls. In a routine evaluation of a patient with hypertension, an echocardiogram is not indicated, and most insurance companies will not pay for this type of imaging as part of an evaluation of a hypertensive patient unless a special reason exists. Furthermore, the physical examination, electrocardiogram, and chest X ray can often establish the diagnosis without the need for an echocardiogram.

84 What Is a TIA, and How Is It Treated?

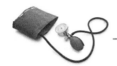

A TIA (transient ischemic attack) is a temporary decrease in the blood supply to a portion of the brain. Often this event is the forerunner of a stroke. Indeed, a TIA is actually a small stroke that can affect speech and the movement of extremities, and it can sometimes lead to a temporary loss of vision in one eye. These spells usually last for less than ten minutes, followed by complete recovery. TIAs probably occur when small thrombi (clots) break off from atherosclerotic plaques (damaged lining of arteries) in the neck or heart and temporarily block small arteries supplying blood to the area of the brain that controls speech, movements of extremities, or vision.

Many, but not all, patients with TIAs are hypertensive. If they are, their blood pressures should be reduced gradually. Medical treatment includes aspirin, which prevents the formation of little thrombi, or warfarin (Coumadin), which is a different kind of blood thinner and a stronger anticoagulant than

> *A TIA (transient ischemic attack) is a transient decrease of blood supply to a portion of the brain.*

aspirin. Sometimes it is necessary to surgically remove a plaque (which is composed mainly of cholesterol and causes obstruction) in the carotid artery of the neck. Treating hypertension will reduce the risk of TIAs and major strokes.

85 What Is a Stroke?

A stroke is a blockage or rupture of an artery in the brain, leading to destruction of the surrounding area of the brain. The result may be paralysis of one or more extremities, difficulty or inability to talk, or disturbed vision, depending upon which area of the brain is involved. Approximately 75 percent of all strokes occur in hypertensive people, so treating high blood pressure can markedly reduce the risk of stroke and death.

A blockage of an artery in the brain may occur in several different ways. For example, a brain artery may become blocked because of atherosclerosis (damage of the lining of an artery from deposits of cholesterol) and a clot formation within the artery. Alternatively, a cholesterol plaque may break off from a carotid artery in the neck or from the aorta and be carried by the bloodstream to an artery in the brain, which it then blocks. In addition, blood clots may form in the left atrium of the heart because of an irregularity of the heart rhythm, known as atrial fibrillation, and can similarly be carried to the brain. It is noteworthy that recent evidence indicates that obesity, even without hypertension, can also cause the heart to enlarge and develop atrial fibrillation.

> A stroke is a blockage or rupture of an artery in the brain, leading to destruction of the surrounding area of the brain. Treating high blood pressure can markedly reduce the risk of stroke and death.

Strokes may sometimes be prevented by surgery intended to prevent atherosclerotic plaques from reaching the brain. Your doctor may recommend low-dose aspirin to prevent many types of stroke or warfarin (Coumadin, an anticoagulant) to prevent formation of blood clots in the heart and reduce the chance of an embolus (clot) traveling to the brain, especially if you have experienced a heart attack or have atrial fibrillation.

86 What Is a Vascular Aneurysm? Can It Be Caused by Hypertension, and How Can It Be Detected and Treated?

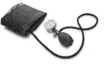

An aneurysm is an abnormal dilation or a bulge in a portion of a blood vessel. It usually results from a weakness in the wall of an artery or the aorta (the largest artery in the body, which carries blood from the heart to arteries supplying blood throughout the body). Hypertension can cause aneurysms to enlarge and rupture; the ensuing hemorrhage can result in extensive damage to surrounding tissue and severe blood loss, which may be fatal.

The weakness of the wall of an artery or aorta usually results from atherosclerosis (hardening and damaging of the artery with deposits of cholesterol on the lining of the vessel); however, perhaps 20 percent of aneurysms are hereditary — the result of a genetic abnormality that weakens the artery wall.

> *A vascular aneurysm is an abnormal dilation or a bulge in a portion of a blood vessel. It usually results from a weakness in the wall of an artery or the aorta.*

These hereditary aneurysms sometimes occur in the brain, where they are called "berry" aneurysms, because they resemble a sac in the shape of a berry. Some aneurysms are associated with an abnormal constriction or narrowing of the aorta known as a coarctation. Coarctations block the flow of blood, causing hypertension in the upper portion of the body and increasing the risk of hemorrhage from any coexisting aneurysms exposed to this increased blood pressure; pressure beyond the constriction in the lower portion of the body and in the legs is less than it is in the upper portion of the body (see Question 38). Hereditary aneurysms of the aorta are sometimes associated with congenital heart disease, and a very small percentage of aneurysms are caused by syphilis or traumatic injuries to blood vessels.

Approximately 75 percent of aortic aneurysms occur in the lower part of the abdomen and result from atherosclerosis. These aneurysms are most prevalent in the elderly, particularly in those with hypertension, and they tend to increase in size with aging. Although they do not generally produce symptoms, they may become painful and tender, and they may cause pain in the abdomen and back as they enlarge. Sometimes these aneurysms may cause very severe pain because of a tear in the aorta, which may lead to a fatal hemorrhage if it ruptures. Often an abdominal aortic aneurysm is detected by a physician as a palpable, pulsatile, non-tender mass in the abdomen; the diagnosis can be confirmed by imaging studies such as an ultrasound, a CAT scan, or an MRI. The five-year risk of rupture with aneurysms less than 2 inches in diameter is 1 to 2 percent, whereas 20 to 40 percent of larger aneurysms will rupture within five years. Therefore, surgical repair with a graft is indicated for large aneurysms. Today, endovascular stenting (a metal device inserted into a blood vessel to keep blood flowing through the vessel) may frequently replace surgery. Beta-blocking drugs are recommended for smaller aneurysms, because these agents reduce the strength of pulsations against the weakened aneurysmal wall and prevent further enlargement. Of course, it is crucial to reduce any elevated blood pressure to 130/80 mm Hg or less in the case of abdominal aneurysm.

Aneurysms located elsewhere in the body may be identified by various imaging techniques and can be treated surgically, if indicated. Aneurysms in the brain may require a clipping procedure or a new surgical technique that places a coil in the aneurysm to obliterate it in order to prevent rupture and hemorrhage in the future.

Of paramount importance in avoiding possible rupture of an aneurysm is a normalization of blood pressure with the administration of appropriate antihypertensive medication.

87 Do Hypertension, High Cholesterol, Obesity, and Diabetes Mellitus Often Go Together? How Do You Treat This Metabolic Syndrome?

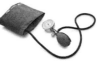

The constellation of (1) hypertension; (2) abnormal blood fats, namely high LDL cholesterol (low-density lipoprotein, the "bad" cholesterol), low HDL (high-density lipoprotein, the "good" cholesterol), and high triglycerides (another "bad" fat); (3) central (upper-body) obesity; and (4) insulin resistance (a decreased ability of insulin to metabolize and store sugar in muscle) and sometimes adult-onset diabetes mellitus has been correctly designated "the deadly quartet" and is now usually called "metabolic syndrome." Left untreated, this set of risk factors will often lead to severe vascular damage, resulting in heart attack, stroke, heart and kidney failure, damage to the eyes with visual impairment, the weakening and rupture of blood vessels, impairment of blood flow to the lower extremities, and death.

> The constellation of hypertension, abnormal blood fats, central (upper-body) obesity, and insulin resistance/diabetes mellitus has been correctly designated "the deadly quartet."

Although the cause of insulin resistance remains poorly understood, this condition is known to be associated with the development of obesity and may be aggravated by excess alcohol consumption. It is the underlying abnormality that leads to adult-onset diabetes mellitus, in which an increased blood concentration of insulin occurs in an effort to compensate for the resistance to insulin metabolism of sugar. (In childhood diabetes, insulin levels in the blood are very low or absent.) Insulin resistance affects approximately 20 percent of the U.S. population and is almost always associated with cardiovascular risk factors, including obesity, abnormal blood fats, hypertension, and salt sensitivity. Whether insulin plays a role in causing hypertension is unclear.

There is no easy way of testing for insulin resistance, but the presence of other findings in the constellation of abnormalities mentioned earlier indirectly establishes its diagnosis. Treatment is directed at achieving the following goals:

- reducing blood pressure to less than 130/80 mm Hg
- reducing body weight, if indicated, by decreasing caloric intake with a low-cholesterol and low-saturated fat diet, and increasing caloric expenditure with appropriate aerobic exercise
- using a low-salt diet — that is, no more that 6 grams (one teaspoonful of sodium chloride), equivalent to 2,400 mg of sodium per day

- limiting daily alcohol consumption to only one or two drinks of spirits, wine, or beer
- quitting smoking
- controlling diabetes, if present

When antihypertensive medication is indicated, it should include an ACE or angiotensin inhibitor, as these drug classes are particularly effective in preventing or minimizing the renal damage that is especially likely to occur in diabetics. For those patients requiring more than one drug, which is usually the case, diuretics (water pills) can prove valuable, as diabetics are frequently salt sensitive and suffer from fluid retention. Finally, low-dose aspirin is recommended after the blood pressure is controlled.

88 What Foods or Drinks Should I Avoid if I Have Hypertension?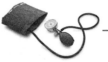

Excess intake of calories, fat, salt, and alcohol, and inadequate intake of potassium may play roles in the development and severity of hypertension.

If you have hypertension and are overweight, it is very important that you make a strong effort to reduce the number of calories in your diet. For most hypertensives who are overweight, weight loss is usually the most effective way of lowering blood pressure. Motivation is essential to dieting success, of course, and we recommend reducing dietary fat to no more that 30 percent of your daily calories. This consideration is important: One gram of fat equals 9 calories, whereas 1 gram of protein or carbohydrate is equivalent to only 4 calories. For this reason, excessive consumption of fat should be avoided to reduce and maintain appropriate weight. Furthermore, limiting saturated fat and cholesterol in the diet is especially important if the LDL (low-density lipoprotein, the "bad" cholesterol) is elevated or the HDL (high-density lipoprotein, the "good" cholesterol) is low, as these conditions may hasten the development and progression of atherosclerosis (hardening of arteries). Reducing caloric intake also depends on reducing the amount of food consumed. Perhaps the most acceptable way of accomplishing this goal is to decrease the portion size rather than to introduce a new, bland diet that the patient does not find palatable.

Curtailing the use of sodium chloride (table salt) is particularly important in salt-sensitive individuals — and an estimated 50 to 60 percent of primary hypertensives are salt sensitive. These individuals may retain excess salt and water and develop hypertension. It is easy to limit excess salt in cooking and to avoid use of the salt shaker. Because 70 to 75 percent of salt is ordinarily consumed in processed foods, however, one should be constantly aware of the of sodium content as indicated on the labels of various foods purchased in supermarkets or elsewhere (see Question 34). Note that some drinks and juices (such as Gatorade, tomato juice, and V8 juice) contain significant amounts of sodium; look for low-sodium versions of the regular products. It is recommended that no more than 6 grams of salt (about one teaspoonful), equivalent to 2,400 mg of sodium, should be ingested daily.

Diets high in potassium (due to the consumption of large amounts of fruits and vegetables) appear to slowly lower blood pressure. This mineral also protects against stroke, replaces some of the excess sodium in the body, and causes sodium to be excreted in the urine.

Of significant importance is the avoidance of excess alcohol in patients with primary hypertension. Excessive alcohol consumption is reportedly responsible for elevated blood pressure in 7 to 10 percent of all hypertensive individuals. Men with hypertension should limit their intake to no more than two usual-sized drinks (spirits, wine, or beer) per day, and women with hypertension should limit alcohol consumption to only one drink daily.

Excessive ingestion of certain kinds of licorice is also known to elevate blood pressure. Licorice contains glycyrrhetinic acid, which causes sodium retention, potassium excretion, and the development of hypertension. Licorice extracts are also present in chewing tobacco, so this product should be avoided. In addition, certain food supplements (for example, those containing ephedrine or yohimbine) should be avoided, as they can constrict the arterioles and cause hypertension. If caffeine-containing drinks cause you to experience excess elevations of blood pressure, it would be wise to switch to decaffeinated brands, especially if you have hypertension. Grapefruit juice can inhibit an enzyme that metabolizes some of the calcium-channel blockers and certain other drugs, causing concentrations of the drugs to build up in the blood and exert a stronger effect in lowering blood pressure; however, significant enzyme inhibition occurs only when large amounts of grapefruit juice are consumed.

Finally, a word of caution about "health foods." Some supplements and herbal remedies may possibly interact with some antihypertensive medications. For example, ginseng may elevate blood pressure and ma huang may cause stroke, heart attack, and sudden death (see Questions 71 and 73). You should always consult your physician before taking food supplements!

89 Why Is My Cholesterol Elevated? Should I Try to Lower It, and What Is a Desirable Level?

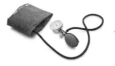

Blood cholesterol may be elevated because of excessive consumption of cholesterol and fat (some of which is converted to cholesterol). Note, however, that 75 percent of cholesterol is produced by the liver (a function that is determined by your genes). Lowering an elevated blood level of cholesterol through use of diet and medications may protect you from hardening of the arteries, heart attack, and stroke.

Total blood cholesterol for adults thirty years or older is considered normal if it is 200 mg or less. In adults twenty-nine years or younger and in adolescents, this level should be about 180 mg or less. Vegetarians usually have total cholesterol levels that are very low, often less than 150 mg.

Even a diet that contains very little cholesterol and fat may not normalize blood cholesterol levels if your liver inappropriately produces too much of this substance. Normally, increased consumption of cholesterol and saturated fat increases blood cholesterol, which is recognized by receptors (structures on liver cells that sense the blood level of cholesterol). Cholesterol in

> *Total blood cholesterol for adults thirty years or older is considered normal if it is 200 mg or less. In adults twenty-nine years or younger and in adolescents, this level should be 180 mg or less.*

the blood attaches to these receptors, enters the liver cells, and then suppresses the production of cholesterol by the liver. If the number of these receptors is decreased, less cholesterol can enter the liver cells and the liver provides less suppression of cholesterol production. As a consequence, levels of cholesterol in the blood become more elevated. Tragically, children in some families inherit few (if any) of these receptors, leading them to develop extremely high cholesterol levels; these children usually die at very young ages from heart attacks. Fortunately, this familial condition is extremely rare.

Cholesterol in the blood consists of the following three major components, which are carried in the blood as lipoproteins:

- low-density lipoprotein (LDL)
- very-low-density lipoprotein (VLDL)
- high-density lipoprotein (HDL)

The main lipoproteins in the blood are LDL and HDL. "Density" simply indicates the weight of these lipoproteins.

LDL is known as "bad" cholesterol, because it can lead to deposits of cholesterol (plaques) on the lining of blood vessels. Plaque formation can block arteries and cause heart attacks and strokes. The desirable level of LDL cholesterol is 100 mg or less.

Slightly higher levels are acceptable if you have no other risk factors (that is, diabetes, cigarette smoking, evidence of coronary heart disease, hypertension, low levels of HDL, or a family history of premature heart attacks). If you have evidence of heart disease, it is always desirable to keep the level of LDL cholesterol below 100 mg.

90 What Is the Story on "Good" and "Bad" Cholesterol and Triglycerides? Can Cholesterol Cause Hypertension?

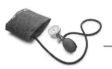

HDL (high-density lipoprotein) is known as the "good" cholesterol because it removes LDL (low-density lipoprotein), or the "bad" cholesterol, from the arteries and carries it to the liver where it is excreted in the bile. Desirable levels of HDL are 45 mg or higher. In general, the higher the level of HDL, the lower the risk of heart disease. In addition, the ratio of total cholesterol to HDL appears be one indicator of risk for heart disease. An acceptable total cholesterol/HDL ratio is roughly 4.5 or less for men and 3.5 or less for women. LDL/HDL ratios are sometimes used to assess the risk of heart disease but are no more accurate than total cholesterol/HDL ratios in this respect.

> *Desirable levels of HDL are 45 mg or higher. An acceptable total cholesterol/HDL ratio is roughly 4.5 or less for men and 3.5 or less for women.*

HDL levels may be increased by appropriate weight loss, aerobic exercise, some antihypertensive medications (alpha blockers), some drugs that are used to lower cholesterol and triglycerides (niacin, statins, and fibrates), the consumption of modest amounts of alcohol, and quitting cigarette smoking. Estrogen may lower LDL and triglycerides and raise HDL, but its use should only be considered in postmenopausal women with a strong family history of cardiovascular disease. Conversely, HDL levels may be decreased by obesity, a lack of exercise, the use of some antihypertensive drugs (beta blockers), and smoking.

Very strong evidence shows that populations that consume high amounts of animal fats and dairy products have a high incidence of death from coronary heart disease, whereas those that consume diets high in fruits, vegetables, fish, and fat from olive oil have a much lower incidence of heart disease. Although cholesterol is essential for the production of cell membranes and hormones in the body, excessive amounts of LDL contribute to blood vessel and heart disease, particularly if some of this cholesterol is oxidized (that is, becomes combined with oxygen). Oxidized cholesterol is especially undesirable, as it is taken up by cells lining the arteries and forms plaques in these vessels. Cholesterol-lowering drugs are used to prevent or minimize the damaging effect of excess cholesterol on arteries (see Question 92).

Triglycerides are another form of lipid (fat) that is mainly carried in the blood by VLDL (very-low-density lipoprotein). Levels may be elevated because of a genetic abnormality or because of an environmental influence (such as obesity, excessive fat consumption, diabetes, or excessive alcohol consumption). Triglycerides become especially elevated shortly after you eat a fatty meal. Therefore, their concentration should be measured while the patient is fasting (fasting is not necessary when measuring total cholesterol, HDL, or LDL). Elevated triglycerides appear to be a less-important risk factor for coronary heart disease, but maintaining them at a level of 150 mg or less is desirable.

Maintaining a normal blood concentration of cholesterol and triglycerides is important for preventing arterial damage, which can impair blood flow in the vessels of the heart, brain, and legs and result in heart attacks, stroke, and pain in the legs when walking. According to some reports, a 1 percent decline in a person's cholesterol level can reduce the risk of death from heart attack by 2 percent. The presence of coronary heart disease calls for intensive efforts to reduce LDL cholesterol and increase HDL cholesterol, if possible. Hypertension in the presence of an elevated LDL level compounds the problem, further accelerating vascular damage and therefore increasing the risk of heart attack and stroke. If lifestyle modifications do not normalize blood pressure and adequately reduce LDL cholesterol, then appropriate drug therapies are indicated. An elevated cholesterol level does not cause hypertension, but it may produce hardening of the arteries, which can then result in systolic hypertension and cause stroke and both heart and kidney diseases.

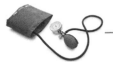

91 What Drugs Are Available to Treat Elevated Blood Cholesterol and Triglycerides? How Do They Work, and What Are Their Side Effects?

Several classes of drugs are effective in lowering cholesterol and triglycerides, both of which are types of lipids (fats) found in the blood. These include niacin (nicotinic acid), bile acid binding resins, fibrates, statins, and other drugs that limit the absorption of cholesterol by the intestines. Table 11 describes their mechanisms of action and side effects.

Table 11. Medications Used to Lower LDL Cholesterol and Triglycerides and to Increase HDL Cholesterol

Drug	Mechanism of Action	LDL	Triglycerides	HDL	Side Effects
Niacin (Niaspan)	Unknown	↓	↓	↑↑	Flushing, itching, fatigue, blurred vision, elevated blood sugar, indigestion, peptic ulcer flare up, liver inflammation
Resins (Questran Colestid)	Bind with bile acids and prevent reabsorption of cholesterol from intestine	↓	None	None	Constipation, indigestion, nausea

Effects on (spans LDL, Triglycerides, HDL columns)

(cont'd.)

Table 11. Medications Used to Lower LDL Cholesterol and Triglycerides and to Increase HDL Cholesterol (cont'd.)

Drug	Mechanism of Action	Effects on			Side Effects
		LDL	Triglyc-erides	HDL	
Fibrates (Lopid, Tricor)	Uncertain, but decreases production of triglycerides by liver and decreases VLDL, which carries triglycerides in blood	↓	↓↓	↑↑	Indigestion, rash. May increase effectiveness of anticoagulants and drugs that lower blood sugar. May interact with statins and cause muscle damage, gallstones, and kidney failure.
Statins [Baycol (cerivastatin), Crestor (rosuvastatin), Lescol (fluvastatin), Lipitor (atorvastatin), Mevacor (lovastatin), Pravachol (pravastatin) Zocor (simvastatin)]	Inhibit HMG-CoA reductase, decrease production of cholesterol by the liver, and increase its removal from the blood	↓↓	↓	(↑)	Increased liver enzymes, rash, itching, headache, muscle pains, and damage accompanied by kidney failure. May interact with fibrates and cause muscle damage.
Zetia (ezetimibe)	Inhibits cholesterol absorption In the intestine	↓	↓	(↑)	Very rare upper respiratory infection, arthralgias, and fatigue. Should not be used in patients with liver disease.

Key: ↑ increase; ↑↑ considerable increase; (↑) may sometimes increase slightly ↓ decrease; ↓↓ considerable decrease; None – no change; ↑↓ variable effect

Note: Regular consumption of Benecol may lower LDL cholesterol by up to 14 percent in people with elevated cholesterol. This margarinelike compound contains a plant substance, sitostanol, that inhibits cholesterol absorption from the intestine with no apparent side effects. It is relatively low in calories and sodium and may be a good substitute for butter; however, you should consult your physician before using it during pregnancy.

It may be helpful for you to discuss this table with your doctor.

Drugs that lower elevated blood concentrations of LDL cholesterol (low-density lipoprotein, also known as "bad" cholesterol) can halt the progression of and may even cause some regression of cholesterol plaques that partially obstruct arteries, thereby improving blood flow and reducing the risk of heart attack and death. Therefore, it is extremely important to consider the use of drugs to lower elevated blood cholesterol and triglycerides when dietary and lifestyle changes fail to reduce these lipid levels. Furthermore, it is critical to lower cholesterol and triglyceride levels in the presence of hypertension, as the combination of these two risk factors poses a far more serious health hazard than the presence of either of these risk factors by itself. The existence of other risk factors — such as coronary heart disease, diabetes, a family history of premature death from heart attack or stroke, cigarette smoking, a sedentary lifestyle, and obesity — may compound the problem and necessitate aggressive efforts to control both hypertension and lipid abnormalities.

As noted earlier, elevated cholesterol and triglyceride levels can have damaging effects on the lining of blood vessels. In contrast, high levels of HDL (high-density lipoprotein, also known as "good" cholesterol) may protect against such damage by removing and transporting deposits of cholesterol from plaques in the arteries to the liver. Thus, a drug that effectively lowers both LDL cholesterol and triglycerides, while raising HDL cholesterol, would be especially desirable.

When lifestyle changes (weight reduction, exercise, restriction of fat to 30 percent of daily calories, and reduction of dietary cholesterol) fail to normalize elevated LDL and triglyceride levels, lipid-lowering drugs should be considered. In general, the higher the levels of LDL and triglycerides and the greater the number of risk factors, the more intensive the effort to combat any correctable conditions should be. The important protective role played by elevated HDL levels must also be considered. Women generally have higher levels of HDL than men do, and often these levels are markedly elevated and mainly account for the elevated level of total cholesterol. An elevated total cholesterol level that results from an elevated HDL level obviously requires no treatment.

Desirable levels of total cholesterol, LDL, HDL, and triglycerides were discussed in Question 90. Table 11 on page 180 lists the various drugs available to treat any lipid abnormalities. All of these drugs can reduce the incidence of nonfatal heart attacks as well as death from heart attacks. The medications may cause undesirable side effects, so your physician may not use them with mild lipid abnormalities that can be corrected by lifestyle changes.

When use of these drugs becomes necessary, your physician will probably suggest starting with a statin. Statins work by inhibiting the enzyme that produces cholesterol, so they are very effective in lowering LDL. In addition, they are moderately effective in lowering triglycerides and may sometimes increase HDL by as much as 5 to 10 percent, depending on the particular statin. The statins are generally better tolerated than are other lipid-lowering drugs. Although side effects are infrequent and usually not severe with these agents, levels of liver enzymes may become elevated, indicating some liver toxicity. This effect is usually mild and requires no change in treatment. If the enzyme changes are pronounced, however, it may be necessary to discontinue medication; elevated enzyme levels almost invariably return to normal after the use of a statin ends. Pain in large muscles (myopathy) can occur and may, very rarely, lead to severe muscle damage that, in turn, can cause kidney failure.

Niacin (or nicotinic acid) can lower both LDL and triglyceride levels, and it usually increases HDL levels significantly. The mechanism of action that produces these effects remains unknown. Flushing is the most common and annoying side effect, but this can often be minimized or prevented by the use of a slow-release formulation.

Resins (Questran or Colestid) bind with bile acids, which contain cholesterol, and increase the elimination of cholesterol in the stool. Some patients find them unpalatable, and many complain of constipation and indigestion. Although resins are fairly effective in reducing LDL cholesterol, they have no effect on triglycerides or HDL. Other medications should be taken at least two hours before the consumption of a resin, as the resin may interfere with the other drugs' absorption. More recently, ezetimibe (Zetia) has proven effective in reducing the absorption of cholesterol by the intestine, and it causes few side effects. It is sometimes used with the statins to enhance the effectiveness of lowering cholesterol in the blood.

Fibrates (Lopid and Tricor) are very effective in lowering triglycerides and increasing HDL, but they have variable effect on LDL. The precise mechanism of action for the fibrates remains somewhat unclear, although the drugs are known to decrease the liver's production of triglycerides. These drugs may enhance both the effect of anticoagulants (blood thinners) and the effect of some drugs used to lower blood sugar.

Of the drugs used to control lipid abnormalities, the statins appear most suitable for lowering LDL cholesterol levels; they also sometimes lower triglyceride levels. If side effects prevent a patient from continuing use of the statins, then niacin and the resins are good alternatives. For marked elevations of triglycerides, the fibrates are most effective in normalizing the lipid concentrations; these drugs have little effect on LDL levels, however. Choosing the appropriate drug and its dosage, monitoring liver enzymes, recognizing side effects, and avoiding drug interactions that could cause harm are the responsibility of the physician.

92 Is It Possible to Prevent Coronary Artery Disease and Heart Attacks?

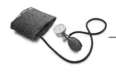

It is very possible to prevent heart disease. The major risk factors for coronary artery disease are hypertension, high levels of cholesterol in the blood, and cigarette smoking. All of these conditions can contribute to hardening of the arteries (atherosclerosis) and subsequent impairment of blood flow to the heart, which can in turn lead to angina (chest pain or a sensation of pressure) and heart attack. Well-conducted clinical trials have confirmed that controlling high blood pressure, controlling high cholesterol, and stopping cigarette smoking markedly reduce a person's risk of coronary heart disease and heart attack. The highest incidence of heart attacks occur in nations whose populations consume the highest amounts of dairy products, saturated fats, and cholesterol. Regular aerobic exercise (see Question 46), if not contraindicated by a physician, may lower elevated blood pressure, aid in maintaining proper weight, elevate "good" cholesterol, and lower "bad" cholesterol, thus preventing or minimizing risk of coronary artery disease. In addition, some preliminary evidence suggests that elevated levels of homocysteine in the blood may be associated with atherosclerosis; therefore, it seems prudent to significantly reduce high homocysteine levels (see Question 94).

Diabetes mellitus is also a major risk factor for atherosclerosis and coronary heart disease. Unfortunately, tight control of the blood sugar of diabetics does not appear to reduce this risk, although this practice does lessen the risk of negative kidney, nerve, and eye complications. If you have diabetes, it is very important that you keep your blood pressure and cholesterol under good control and that you do not smoke cigarettes.

93 If I Am Very Old, Do I Need Treatment for Hypertension or High Cholesterol?

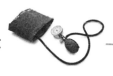

Trials that included patients older than sixty-five years revealed that the benefits of antihypertensive therapy are even greater for older patients than they are for younger patients. This finding probably reflects the fact that older patients are at greater risk for cardiovascular disease than younger patients — hence the benefits from treatment are correspondingly greater. Older patients who receive treatment for their high blood pressure have fewer strokes, fewer heart attacks, and less congestive heart failure than do older patients with untreated hypertension. This relationship also holds true for patients over age eighty.

The benefits of treating elevated "bad" cholesterol (LDL — low-density lipoprotein) with medication in older men, especially in those with low levels of "good" cholesterol (HDL — high density lipoprotein), are fairly well established. On the other hand, less evidence has been gathered to prove any beneficial effects from treating elevated "bad" cholesterol in women at any age. Most women have relatively high levels of the "good" cholesterol in their blood, which protects them from cardiovascular disease until they reach menopause, when they no longer have the protection from naturally occurring estrogens. Reducing significantly elevated levels of triglycerides in the blood is desirable in both men and women. Lifestyle changes are, of course, always recommended when indicated.

> The benefits of treating elevated LDL levels with medication in elderly men, especially in those with low HDL levels, are fairly well established. Less evidence has been gathered to prove beneficial effects from treating elevated "bad" (LDL) cholesterol in women at any age.

94. What Is Homocysteine? Does It Have Harmful Effects, and What Should I Do If I Have an Excess Amount?

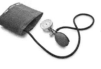

Homocysteine is an amino acid (a substance used by the body to manufacture proteins) that is normally present in your blood. Some concern has arisen that elevated levels of homocysteine in the blood are correlated with damage to blood vessels, hardening of the arteries (atherosclerosis), and an increased risk of heart attack and stroke. Elevations of homocysteine in the blood result in excessive amounts of homocysteine in the urine (homocystein-uria). Children with homocysteinuria due to a hereditary abnormality develop hardening of the arteries as frequently as do older adults. Thus, it appears that elevated homocysteine levels in the blood accelerate the development of atherosclerosis.

Approximately 10 percent of all people have a defective version of the enzyme that ordinarily clears homocysteine from the blood. Such a defect enables abnormally high amounts of homocysteine to become concentrated in the blood. However, the main reason for homocysteine elevations is inadequate consumption of folic acid, vitamin B-6, and vitamin B-12, all of which are found in vegetables (especially lima beans and broccoli). An estimated 40 percent of Americans consume inadequate amounts of folic acid.

> Homocysteine is an amino acid that is normally present in your blood. Some concern has arisen that elevated levels of homocysteine in the blood are correlated with damage to blood vessels, hardening of the arteries, and an increased risk of heart attack and stroke.

Because of the risk and negative complications that result from hardening of the arteries (including heart attacks, strokes, and blood vessel disease), it is recommended that folic acid be taken daily if the homocysteine level in the blood is elevated or the folic acid level is abnormally low. The presence of hypertension could increase the likelihood of negative results related to atherosclerosis if the level of homocysteine is elevated in the blood. Nevertheless, the level of homocysteine in the blood is very rarely measured, as its role in causing hardening of the arteries remains controversial and there is no strong evidence that lowering homocysteine reduces the risks of developing the negative complications related to atherosclerosis.

95 Are High Cholesterol and High Blood Pressure Related?

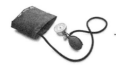

High blood pressure and high blood cholesterol are both recognized as risk factors for heart disease, arterial disease, and stroke, but they act independently of each other. A person can have high blood pressure without high cholesterol, and vice versa. Certainly patients with high blood cholesterol should be checked for hypertension, and individuals with hypertension should be checked for high blood cholesterol, because the combination of the two conditions often go together and represent a powerful risk factor for heart disease and stroke. If high levels of cholesterol in the blood result in hardening of the arteries (atherosclerosis) and hence decreased elasticity of the aorta and large arteries, systolic blood pressure would increase as well.

96 What Are Antioxidants, and Should I Be Taking Them?

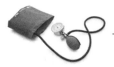

The excitement and interest by both the public and the medical profession in the possible benefits of antioxidants in the prevention of a variety of chronic diseases have been enormous.

> *The antioxidants that have been most extensively evaluated for their therapeutic effects are vitamin E (tocopherol), vitamin C (ascorbic acid), and beta-carotene (which the body converts into vitamin A) and many other carotenoids.*

The antioxidants that have been most extensively evaluated for their therapeutic effects are vitamin E (tocopherol), vitamin C (ascorbic acid), and beta-carotene (which the body converts into vitamin A) and many other carotenoids.

The main sources of antioxidants are fruits and vegetables, although tea and coffee are also a notable source. The National Cancer Institute and the National Research Council recommend that we eat five servings of both fruits and vegetables each day for optimal health, but in reality only a very small percentage of Americans consume these amounts.

Antioxidants act as "scavengers" or "traps" of certain harmful chemicals, thereby preventing or minimizing the harmful effects of the by-products of oxidation that result from normal body metabolism. These harmful by-products consist of "free radicals"—unstable, toxic chemical agents. Some evidence indicates that these free radicals may cause extensive damage to DNA, proteins, carbohydrates, and lipids in cells and tissues; increase cell division; and eventually lead to injury to and the clog-ging of arteries and to the development of cancer. Cigarette smok-ing and ultraviolet radiation are environmental factors that can promote the formation of free radicals.

As yet, however, the value of antioxidants in the treatment or prevention of various diseases has not been established.

The effects of beta-carotene and other carotenoids have been less-extensively studied, and their effectiveness as antioxidants remains unclear. No evidence shows that they have any effect on blood pressure or blood levels of cholesterol. The carotenoids' ability to prevent coronary artery damage, heart disease, and can-cer remains under investigation.

97 Why Is Potassium Important in the Management of Hypertension?

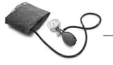

Attention has increasingly been focusing on the importance of dietary potassium in reducing elevated blood pressure. The Die-tary Approaches to Stop Hypertension (DASH) diet, which calls for high amounts of fruits and vegetables (a rich source of potas-sium) and also is low in fat, can lower both systolic and diastolic blood pressure (BP). This diet consists of grains, fruits, vegetables, low-fat or nonfat dairy foods, and limited amounts of meats, poul-try, fish, nuts, seeds, and legumes (see Table 12 on the next page and Question 49).

In one study, the DASH diet reduced fat consumption to ap-proximately 27 percent of the total diet, down from the average fat intake of 37 percent. After eight weeks on this diet, hyperten-sive patients experienced reductions in their systolic and diastolic pressures of 11.4 and 5.5 mm Hg, respectively. This decline oc-curred without any changes in alcohol or salt consumption, or weight loss, any of which by itself might have reduced BP. The DASH diet also lowered the BP of those with borderline elevations, sug-gesting that it may be helpful in preventing hypertension.

Table 12. The DASH Diet (Based on about 2,000 calories per day)

Food Group	Daily Servings	Serving Sizes	Examples	Significance to the DASH diet
Grains and grain products	7–8	1 slice bread ½ cup dry cereal ½ cup cooked rice, pasta, or cereal	Whole-wheat bread, (½) English muffin, (small) pita bread, bagel, cereals, grits, oatmeal (Typical bagel = 4 servings of grains)	Major sources of energy and fiber
Vegetables	4–5	1 cup raw, leafy vegetable ½ cup cooked vegetable 6 oz vegetable juice	Tomatoes, potatoes, carrots, peas, squash, broccoli, turnip greens, collards, kale, spinach, artichokes, beans, sweet potatoes	Rich sources of potassium, magnesium, and fiber
Fruits	4–5	6 oz fruit juice 1 medium fruit ¼ cup dried fruit ½ cup fresh, frozen, or canned fruit	Apricots, bananas, dates, oranges, grapefruit, mangoes, melons, peaches, pineapples, prunes, raisins, strawberries, tangerines	Important sources of potassium, magnesium, and fiber
Low-fat or nonfat dairy foods	2–3	8 oz milk 1 cup yogurt 1½ oz cheese	Skim or 1-percent milk, skim or low-fat buttermilk, nonfat or low-fat yogurt, part-skim mozzarella cheese, nonfat cheese	Major sources of calcium and protein
Meats, poultry, fish	2 or less	3 oz cooked meats, poultry, or fish	Select only lean meat; trim away visible fats; broil, roast, or boil instead of frying; remove skin from poultry (can also grill)	Rich sources of protein and magnesium
Eggs*	No more than 6 each week			

(cont'd.)

Table 12. The DASH Diet (Based on about 2,000 calories per day) (cont'd.)

Food Group	Daily Servings	Serving Sizes	Examples	Significance to the DASH diet
Nuts, seeds, legumes	4–5 per week	1½ oz or ⅓ cup nuts, ½ oz or 2 Tbsp seeds, ½ cup cooked legumes	(Unsalted) almonds, filberts, mixed nuts, peanuts, walnuts, sunflower seeds, lentils, kidney beans	Rich sources of energy, magnesium, potassium, protein, and fiber
Fats and oils	2–3	1 tsp soft margarine, vegetable oil, or butter, 1 Tbsp regular fat mayonnaise or salad dressing, 2 Tbsp low fat or nonfat salad dressing or mayonnaise	Soft margarine, low-fat mayonnaise, light salad dressing, vegetable oil, (such as corn, canola, olive, or safflower)	Source of essential fatty acids, minor source of energy
Sweets	5 per week	1 Tbsp sugar 1 Tbsp jelly or jam ½ oz jelly beans 8 oz lemonade	Maple syrup, sugar, jelly, jam, fruit-flavored gelatin, jelly beans, hard candy, fruit punch, sorbet, ices	Sweets should be low in fat. Minor source of energy

(Source: "Dietary Approaches to Stop Hypertension" (DASH). *Sixth Report of the Joint National Committee on Prevention, Detection, Evaluation, and Treatment of High Blood Pressure* (November 1997). [The DASH Diet—NIH publication 01-4082. Revised May 2001.] Slight modifications in parentheses for clarity.)

* Added eggs to the DASH diet. Note: no more than six eggs per week; egg whites do not have to be limited. People with diabetes or high LDL cholesterol should consume eggs only occasionally, and no more than once per week.

Potassium apparently replaces and eliminates excess sodium from body tissues, which reduces BP levels in humans and animals with salt-sensitive hypertension. Potassium also dilates the blood vessels. It is noteworthy that such supplements lower BP more dramatically in hypertensive individuals than they do in non-hypertensive subjects; this antihypertensive

Potassium apparently replaces and eliminates excess sodium from body tissues, which reduces blood pressure in humans and animals with salt-sensitive hypertension.

effect on systolic and diastolic BP is more pronounced in subjects on a high-salt diet.

Diets high in potassium may protect against stroke. An increase in daily potassium intake of even one serving of fresh fruits or vegetables was associated with a 40 percent reduction in the risk of stroke!

Of seminal interest was the extraordinary finding reported approximately twenty-five years ago by Dr. Louis Tobian and his associates — namely, that dietary potassium can almost totally prevent stroke in stroke-prone rats with hypertension and in salt-induced hypertensive rats. In contrast, a very high percentage of rats with similar levels of hypertension but receiving a low-potassium diet died from strokes. The explanation of how potassium prevents strokes is not clear.

Our own experimental research on salt-sensitive rats has shed some new light on this subject and probably best explains how potassium prevents strokes and kidney damage in rats. In our investigation, consuming a liberal amount of dietary potassium considerably reduced BP and markedly improved the circulation to the brain and kidney. This return of the circulation toward the normal pattern appears to prevent strokes and minimize damage to the kidneys. Similar changes may occur in humans with salt-sensitive hypertension; confirming this notion, however, requires further studies. The bottom line is that consumption of foods rich in potassium, especially fruits and vegetables, may both lower BP and reduce the occurrence of stroke. It is also conceivable that a potassium-rich diet may minimize the development of hypertension in individuals with borderline elevations of BP.

Greater consumption of foods rich in potassium appears to have no harmful effects in normal subjects. In some individuals with kidney disease or in patients taking antihypertensive drugs that retain potassium (such as ACE inhibitors, angiotensin receptor blockers, and potassium-sparing diuretics), intake of large amounts of potassium through diet, medications, or salt substitutes may cause dangerous elevations of potassium in the blood that can create a serious disturbance in the heart rhythm and even cardiac arrest.

Nevertheless, fruits and vegetables should be consumed very frequently by most people. This recommendation is especially important for African Americans, who tend to eat relatively small amounts of fruits and vegetables and have a particularly high occurrence of hypertension, stroke, and kidney failure.

98 Are Calcium and Magnesium Important in the Management of Hypertension, and Should I Add Them to My Diet?

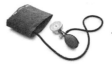

Calcium is important to many bodily functions, including muscle contraction, bone formation, blood clotting, hormone and enzyme activity, and the functioning of cell membranes. Some reports indicate that a low calcium intake is responsible for elevations in blood pressure (BP) and that increasing dietary calcium may lower BP. The results of increasing dietary calcium or using calcium supplements to lower BP have been disappointing. Consequently, use of calcium to lower BP is not advised.

Adequate consumption of calcium is important in the prevention of osteoporosis (a condition in which bones lose calcium, making them brittle and easy to fracture). Bone density can be measured radiographically to determine the existing degree of osteoporosis.

> To date, the results of increasing dietary calcium or using calcium supplements to lower blood pressure have been disappointing. Consequently, use of calcium to lower blood pressure is not advised.

Although it is recommended that individuals younger that sixty-five years of age consume 1,000 mg of calcium daily and that those older than sixty-five consume 1,500 mg daily, this goal is rarely achieved by diet alone. Fat-free and low-fat dairy products (milk, cheese, yogurt), canned fish with bones, some vegetables (navy beans, turnips, broccoli), and many foods that are fortified with calcium (and often vitamin D) are excellent and healthy sources of this mineral. Calcium absorption from the intestine is enhanced by vitamin D, which should also be added to the diet if the patient shows evidence of osteoporosis. Supplemental calcium is available in a variety of tablets; antacids such as Rolaids and Tums contain approximately 500 mg per tablet and can be used as a source of calcium. It is preferable to use a calcium citrate supplement that does not require acid in the stomach for optimal absorption; this type of pill can then be taken any time during the day.

Some people have questioned whether the calcium-channel blockers used to lower BP could interfere with bodily functions other than dilating arteries, slowing heart rate, and exerting beneficial effects on heart-muscle function. In fact, these drugs do not significantly alter function elsewhere in the body. In particular, they do not affect calcium metabolism in bone or influence the development or treatment of osteoporosis. Long-acting thiazide diuretics (water pills) used to lower BP, on the other hand, cause retention of calcium by the body, which would tend to benefit patients with osteoporosis. Loop diuretics have the opposite effect, promoting loss of calcium from the body.

One word of caution: Taking megadoses (very large amounts) of calcium and vitamin D can be very toxic and result in the development of kidney stones and damage to the kidneys. More is not necessarily better!

Magnesium is even less effective in lowering BP than is calcium. No good evidence suggests that this mineral can decrease BP, so no reason exists to give magnesium supplements unless the patient has a magnesium deficit. Magnesium plays an important role in the action of enzymes, cell membrane function, and protein metabolism, and it may block calcium channels. It is recommended that men and women consume 350 mg a day and

265 mg a day, respectively. Good sources of magnesium include green leafy vegetables, whole grains, meats, poultry, fish, seeds, nuts, and water.

A healthy diet should contain the recommended amounts of calcium and magnesium, but administration of these minerals as supplements does not offer a significant benefit in the treatment of hypertension.

99 What Causes Low Blood Pressure, and Is It Harmful? What Are the Symptoms of Low Blood Pressure, in Case My Medication Is Excessive?

In general, it can be said that "the lower the blood pressure (BP) the better" — as long as the individual does not have any symptoms of low blood pressure (see Question 77). This statement is true because the risks of heart attack and stroke are lower when BP remains at a relatively low level.

For many years, a systolic BP of 140 mm Hg and a diastolic pressure of 90 mm Hg were considered normal. Elevations above these levels were designated as hypertension, and they were associated with an increased chance of stroke, heart attack, heart and kidney failure, and impaired vision. It is true that the frequency of these negative complications increases as blood pressure becomes more elevated. More recently, however, physicians have recognized that the chance of these complications progressively decreases as BP becomes significantly lower than 140/90 mm Hg. Optimal BP levels appear to be about 120/80 mm Hg. Many normal young women, especially those who are underweight and have thin arms, have blood pressures of 90/60 mm Hg or slightly less without demonstrating any symptoms suggesting that their pressures are too low. It is also normal for BP in the first, and especially in the second, trimester of pregnancy to decrease below the normal BP levels of nonpregnant women.

Abnormally low blood pressure, known as hypotension, may result when a person stands (postural hypotension) if some defect in sympathetic nerve activity causes an impairment of the constriction of blood vessels; such a nerve-related defect may occur with diabetes, some diseases of the nervous system, and certain adrenal gland tumors. Other causes of hypotension include severe dehydration, blood loss, and allergic reactions. Various types of heart disease (especially those causing rate and rhythm disturbances) can cause a sudden, momentary drop in BP. A particularly common type of sudden drop in BP, which occurs more frequently in young individuals, is due to a vasovagal reflex (a simple faint). This reflex of the nervous system dilates blood vessels and slows the heart rate, thereby leading to a dramatic decline in BP. This condition may result from sudden anxiety and fear or from an emotionally upsetting experience, such as the sight of blood. It does not result from a disease or disability — even the most stout of heart may experience a fall in blood pressure with loss of consciousness! In addition, overmedication with drugs that lower BP can cause hypotension, with the BP drop being particularly apt to occur when the patient is in the standing position.

> Abnormally low blood pressure, known as hypotension, may result when a person stands (*postural hypotension*) *if* some defect in sympathetic nerve activity causes an impairment of the constriction of blood vessels. Hypotension may also result from severe dehydration, blood loss, allergic reactions, heart disease, vasovagal reflex, or overmedication with blood-pressure-lowering drugs.

Hypotension is usually accompanied by faintness, lightheadedness, unsteadiness, and a rapid heartbeat. In some instances, mental confusion, impaired vision, and a temporary loss of consciousness may occur, which, of course, may result in a fall and serious injury. Chronic fatigue is not a symptom of hypotension.

Postural hypotension is more apt to occur in older and frail people, especially if they are inactive or bedridden. For this reason, older patients are often started on lower doses of antihypertensive drugs than are younger and more robust individuals. It is important that older patients on antihypertensive medication take extra time in getting out of bed during the night and when arising in the morning. Sitting on the side of the bed for a minute or two and then holding onto something stable (such as a chair or table) may permit these individuals' vascular systems and BP to better adjust to the posture change, thereby preventing symptoms of hypotension and loss of consciousness.

A special warning should be given to all patients who take alpha-blocking drugs (such as Minipress, Hytrin, Cardura), as these medications block the sympathetic nerves from causing blood vessel constriction. This constriction normally occurs upon standing and prevents blood from pooling in the legs due to the effect of gravity. A small percentage of patients will experience a marked drop in BP when they stand up after taking their first dose of an alpha blocker (see Question 66). The good news is that marked postural hypotension does not continue with subsequent use of these drugs, although caution is still advised when the dose of the drug is increased.

Commonly used antihypertensive drugs typically do not cause a marked, sudden drop in BP. The ability of some of the short-acting calcium-channel blockers (such as Procardia) to cause a rapid drop in BP is undesirable and potentially dangerous, as the resulting hypotension can significantly decrease the blood supply to the heart and brain and possibly produce a heart attack or stroke. For this reason, short-acting calcium-channel blockers are no longer used to treat hypertension.

Some antihypertensive drugs reduce BP more rapidly than others do. If you take antihypertensive drugs and experience light-headedness or feel you are going to faint, you should immediately sit or (preferably) lie down, as this position should reduce the effect of postural hypotension and improve the circulation to the brain. To document whether your lightheadedness or faint feeling is due to postural hypotension caused by your antihypertensive medication, it is essential to determine whether a pronounced drop in BP occurs when you change from a recumbent or seated position to a standing position. Consult your physician immediately if you experience symptoms of hypotension so that your medication can be adjusted, if necessary.

Finally, it should be mentioned that patients with angina (pain in the chest due to insufficient blood supply to the heart) who are taking nitrates (e.g., nitroglycerine) to control the pain may develop hypotension if they also take drugs that produce nitric oxide (e.g., Viagra, Cialis, Levitra). The latter drugs will further increase dilation of blood vessels caused by nitrates and can produce very low blood pressure levels that could cause a patient to fall and be injured and possibly result in a heart attack.

100 How Can I Help Prevent Hypertension in My Children?

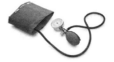

As mentioned previously (see Question 33), there is a strong genetic link to the development of hypertension. However, behavioral factors, especially excess weight gain, excessive salt consumption (particularly in people who are salt sensitive), and inadequate physical activity are even more important than genetics, and parents can play a key role in influencing the lifestyle of their children. Environmental and social circumstances can, of course, play a role in influencing behavior. As the humanitarian Dr. Albert Schweitzer said, "Example is not the main thing in influencing others. It is the *only* thing."

Of special concern is the obesity crisis in America and many other parts of the world. The major negative complications that occur due to obesity (hypertension, type 2 diabetes, abnormalities in blood fats [cholesterol and triglycerides], many cancers, and sleep apnea) cause up to 300,000 deaths in the United States annually and cost the nation $147 billion dollars each year. Weight gain increases the chance and severity of these negative complications. About 50 percent of obese Americans have hypertension, and being overweight or obese is increasing remarkably in children, and their blood pressure is rising. Furthermore, it is anticipated that 30 percent of Caucasians and 50 percent of African Americans and Hispanics born in 2000 will develop diabetes during their lifetime if obesity continues to escalate in our nation, and it is possible that parents will live longer than their children.

Decreasing the portion size of meals, avoiding large amounts of saturated fat, and limiting sugar in food and drinks — coupled with appropriate physical activity — will help our children, just as it helps us, to maintain a normal body weight and physical fitness.

Kidney damage resulting from diabetes or impaired blood flow to the kidneys caused by deposits of cholesterol with hardening (atherosclerosis) of the arteries to the kidneys may also cause hypertension. Sleep apnea, usually the result of obesity, can also cause hypertension.

Finally, excess salt consumption is a major cause of hypertension, which afflicts about 72 million Americans. It is reported that there would be 150,000 fewer deaths each year if Americans would decrease their salt consumption by 50 percent!

The food consumed by parents is often the food consumed by their children. Also, how much physical activity parents engage in often influences the amount of physical activity undertaken by their children. Therefore, healthy nutrition — especially the DASH (Dietary Approaches to Stop Hypertension) eating plan, which promotes eating lots of fruits and vegetables, low-fat or nonfat dairy products, lean meat, poultry (without the skin), fish, grains, nuts, legumes and limiting salt consumption (see Question 34) — has been shown to be effective in preventing hypertension and lowering blood pressure in adults with hypertension. The DASH diet should be helpful for children, too.

People with normal blood pressure should consume no more than 6 grams (a teaspoonful) of salt (about 2,400 mg of sodium) daily; people with hypertension or diabetes should consume no more than 3.8 grams of salt (about 1,500 mg of sodium) daily. There are several ways to reduce salt consumption. Substitute herbs, spices, and lemon juice for salt when preparing some foods to improve their taste. It is also wise to remove the salt shaker from the table and to limit salt addition in food preparation. Most important, however, is to carefully read the food labels of processed foods in order to avoid excess salt consumption, since about 75 percent of dietary salt comes from processed foods.

Therefore, to keep blood pressure from rising and to help prevent hypertension in your children, it is extremely important to help them obtain and maintain at a healthy weight, reduce salt intake, and remain physically active. Instilling a healthy lifestyle at a very young age (preschool through second grade), when children are especially willing to listen and learn from adults, appears to be an ideal period to provide effective guidance. Efforts to benefit the health of young children should be continued as they grow older.

101 Where Can I Get Additional and *Reliable* Information about Hypertension and Some of Its Disease Complications?

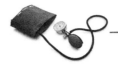

American Heart Association
7272 Greenville Ave.
Dallas TX 75231-4596
www.amhrt.org

American Society of Hypertension, Inc. (ASH)
148 Madison Ave., 5th Fl.
New York NY 10016
(212) 696-9099
www.ash-us.org

Mayo Clinic Health Information
www.mayoclinic.com

National Heart, Lung, and Blood Institute
PO Box 30105
Bethesda MD 20824-0105
Recorded information: (800) 575-9355
www.nhlbi.nih.gov

National Hypertension Association, Inc.
324 E. 30th St.
New York NY 10016
(212) 889-3557
www.nathypertension.org

National Kidney Foundation
30 E. 33rd St.
New York NY 10016
(800) 622-9010
www.kidney.org

National Stroke Association
9707 E. Easter Ln., Ste. B
Centennial CO 80112
(800) 787-6537
www.stroke.org

Hypertension Education Foundation
PO Box 651
Scarsdale NY 10583
www.hypertensionfoundation.org

— Glossary

ACE inhibitor: A drug that lowers blood pressure by inhibiting the angiotensin-converting enzyme (ACE) from producing angiotensin, which constricts arteries and arterioles and elevates blood pressure.

acromegaly: An endocrine disease causing enlargement of parts of the skeleton due to oversecretion of growth hormone by the pituitary gland.

aerobic exercise: Activity requiring motion that increases oxygen consumption, such as walking, running, bicycling, swimming, and other active sports activities.

alcohol dehydrogenase: An enzyme in the digestive tract that metabolizes alcohol.

aldosterone: A hormone from the adrenal gland that causes the kidney to retain sodium and excrete potassium.

alpha₁ blocker: A drug that blocks norepinephrine (a hormone that constricts arterioles) from stimulating receptors on arterioles, thereby causing arterioles to dilate and lowering blood pressure.

alpha₁ receptors: "Targets" on various cells that, when stimulated by norepinephrine (or similar substances), cause a number of responses including constriction of arteries and arterioles, which in turn causes hypertension.

alpha₂ agonist: A drug that acts on the brain to decrease sympathetic nerve activity and thereby lower blood pressure.

anaerobic exercise: Activity requiring minimal motion without much increase in intake of oxygen, such as weight lifting.

anaphylaxis: An allergic reaction, usually to certain insect stings, vaccinations prepared with egg products, or certain foods or drugs that often cause hives, itching, angioedema, and sometimes airway obstruction as well as a marked decrease in blood pressure, which may lead to death.

aneroid sphygmomanometer: A type of sphygmomanometer that measures blood pressure on a dial and that depends on the displacement of a spring rather than a mercury column. This device's accuracy should be compared periodically with results of a mercury sphygmomanometer, as the latter is the most reliable method of measuring blood pressure.

aneurysm: A small or large dilatation, or "ballooning out," in the wall of an artery due to a weakness in that wall.

angina pectoris: A heaviness, pressure, squeezing sensation, or pain in the chest due to insufficient blood supply to the heart. It is usually brought on by exertion or emotional upset and relieved by rest.

angioedema: A vascular reaction usually causing swelling in the skin and/ or upper-respiratory and gastrointestinal tracts.

angioplasty: A technique using a catheter with a balloon that can be in- flated to expand an artery.

angiotensin: A substance in the blood (formed by renin) that is a powerful constrictor of arteries and arterioles.

anticoagulant: Any substance that prevents blood from coagulating (clot- ting).

antihypertensive medications: Drugs that lower elevated blood pressure.

antioxidants: Substances that prevent the harmful oxidation effects of cer- tain chemicals in the body that may cause hardening of the arteries and cancer.

aorta: The largest artery in the body, which carries oxygenated blood pumped from the left muscular chamber of the heart, extends through the chest and abdomen, and branches into arteries supplying blood to the entire body.

apnea: A transient cessation of breathing (occurring during sleep).

arrhythmia: Abnormal heart rhythm or heart rate.

arteries: The vessels that carry blood from the aorta to all parts of the body and end in arterioles, which then are connected to the capillaries.

arterioles: The smallest arteries that carry blood from larger arteries to cap- illaries, which in turn supply tissues with blood. Arterioles have smooth muscle in their walls that permits constriction or dilation, which can raise or lower blood pressure.

arteriosclerosis: A "hardening" of an artery due to thickness of the wall, causing a loss of elasticity.

atherosclerosis: A "hardening" of an artery with deposits of cholesterol and blood cells on the inner lining of the artery, accompanied by the forma- tion of plaques that can partially or totally impede blood flow.

atrial fibrillation: Irregular rapid movements of the atrial muscles without normal contraction to expel blood from the two small chambers of the heart into the ventricles.

atrium: One of a pair of small chambers of the heart that receive blood from the veins and expel it into the ventricles, the pumping chambers of the heart.

beta blocker: A drug that lowers blood pressure mainly by blocking beta receptors on the heart, which slows the heart rate, and in the kidneys, thereby preventing release of renin from the kidneys and inhibiting their production of a substance (angiotensin) that constricts arterioles.

beta receptors: "Targets" on various cells that, when stimulated by epi- nephrine and norepinephrine (or similar substances), cause a number of responses, including those related to an increased rate and strength of heart muscle contraction, which can increase blood pressure.

biofeedback: A technique designed to aid an individual to sense or feel a change in bodily function (e.g., heart rate or blood pressure), which permits the individual to lower his blood pressure and heart rate by control of mental and bodily function (e.g., increased relaxation).

blood pressure: The pressure exerted by the blood against the walls of the arteries.

body mass index (BMI): A measure of ideal and excessive weight; a weight-to-height index calculated by dividing weight in kilograms by the square of height in meters.

brand-name drugs: Drugs named by the manufacturing pharmaceutical company and protected by a patent. Brand-name drugs are more expensive than generic drugs but no more effective.

bruit: A sound or murmur usually heard near or over a narrowed artery and occurring with each heartbeat.

calcium: The most abundant mineral in the body, which is essential for constriction of blood vessels, normal heartbeat, nerve impulses, blood clotting, and many chemical reactions.

calcium-channel blocker: A drug that blocks the entry of calcium into the smooth muscles of arteries and arterioles, thereby preventing their constriction and causing them to dilate, lowering blood pressure. Some of these drugs also depress the rate and pumping force of the heart.

capillaries: Minute vessels connecting arterioles and venules. The capillaries form networks throughout the body tissues that permit exchange of substances between the blood and tissue fluid.

cardiovascular: Involving the heart (cardio) and blood vessels (vascular).

carotene: A substance found in many plants (especially carrots) that is converted into vitamin A in the body.

carotenoids: A group of substances of red or yellow pigment that are found in animal fat and some plants.

CAT (or CT) scan: Meaning "computerized axial tomography," this scan is an X-ray technique that records many images of the body in multiple planes (views).

cessation: Discontinuance.

cholesterol: A fat-like substance (lipid) used especially to build cell membranes and make some hormones. It is present only in animal tissues and dairy products (such as eggs, milk, and butter). Cholesterol is made in the liver and absorbed from food in the intestines. It is transported in the blood mainly as LDL (low-density lipoprotein: the "bad" cholesterol) and HDL (high-density lipoprotein: the "good" cholesterol).

claudication: Pain or fatigue of muscles, particularly experienced in the leg muscles upon walking, that is caused by inadequate circulation and usually results from atherosclerosis of the arteries supplying blood to the muscles. Sometimes referred to as "intermittent claudication," it is induced by walking and is relieved by rest.

coarctation: A congenital, localized constriction or narrowing of the aorta resulting in hypertension in the upper body (above the constriction) and low blood pressure in the lower body (below the constriction).

complications: The results of a disease.

congestive heart failure: Results from diseases or conditions (hypertension, coronary artery disease, myocardial infarction, valvular disease, inflammation, and so on) that impair the pumping efficiency of the heart and cause accumulation of blood and fluid in the lungs and usually elsewhere in the body.

constriction: A narrowing of the caliber: for example, in arteries and arterioles due to contraction of smooth muscle cells. This constriction elevates blood pressure.

contraindication: Any condition that makes a treatment undesirable and inadvisable.

coronary artery disease: Damage of the arteries supplying blood to the heart muscle. This disease is usually the result of cholesterol plaques on the lining of the arteries that impair blood supply and may cause angina (chest pressure or pain) or heart attack.

Cushing's syndrome: A condition caused by either excessive amounts of an adrenal hormone (cortisol) in the blood or excessive administration of a synthetic hormone (corticosteroid), which results in an altered body appearance and often hypertension.

DASH: An acronym for "Dietary Approaches to Stop Hypertension."

diabetes mellitus: A condition causing an elevation of blood sugar due to lack of insulin (type I, occurs in childhood) or resistance to the effect of insulin metabolism (type II, adult onset diabetes).

dialysis (hemodialysis): A method of removing elevated levels of waste products and undesirable chemicals from the blood of patients with severe kidney failure. Blood can be continuously passed through an artificial kidney containing dialyzing fluid, or dialyzing fluid can be continuously introduced into and removed from the peritoneal cavity (abdomen) to "cleanse" the blood and restore it to a more normal composition.

diastole: The period between beats when the heart is at rest and not contracting.

diastolic blood pressure: The pressure between beats when the heart is not contracting; it is the lower of the two numbers recorded as the blood pressure.

diuretic: A drug that causes the kidney to excrete increased amounts of salt and water and lowers blood pressure.

DNA: Deoxyribonucleic acid. This class of nucleic acids, which are found

chiefly in the nucleus of cells, causes transference of genetic characteristics and synthesis of proteins.

doppler ultrasonography: A technique using ultrasound waves to determine blood flow.

echocardiogram: A diagnostic technique utilizing an instrument that is
moved about on the chest and employs sonar (echo) waves to visualize
abnormalities in the anatomy or the function of the heart and its valves.

eclampsia: A serious condition occurring in late pregnancy that follows
preeclampsia, with marked elevation of blood pressure, sometimes con-
vulsive seizures, retention of fluid, and occasionally death of the mother
and fetus.

elaborate: To produce.

elastic recoil of the aorta: The return to the normal caliber of the aorta
after being distended by blood pumped into it from the heart. The return
to normal caliber depends on the "elastic" quality of the aorta.

electrocardiogram (ECG or EKG): A graphic display of the electrical activity of the heart, recorded from electrodes on the chest and extremities.

embolus: A clot brought by the blood from another location where it origi-
nated that obstructs the circulation.

enzyme: A protein that speeds up a chemical reaction.

epinephrine (adrenaline): A hormone from the adrenal gland that can increase the rate and pumping force of the heart, constrict some arterioles,
and dilate other arterioles.

ESRD: End stage renal disease; very severe kidney failure.

essential (primary) hypertension: Primary hypertension accounts for almost 95 percent of the hypertensive population. The cause of this type
of hypertension remains unknown.

fecal: Pertaining to the excrement discharged from the intestine (feces).

fetus: The developing young in the uterus after the second month of pregnancy.

fibromuscular dysplasia: Constriction or constrictions of an artery supplying the kidney that can lead to impaired blood supply to the kidney, with
subsequent release of renin and development of hypertension.

free radical: A damaging chemical, usually an oxidation by-product, that
is thought to damage the lining of arteries and possibly play a role in
causing cancer.

generic drug: A drug that is not protected by a patent. Its name is usually
descriptive of its chemical composition, and the drug is typically less
expensive than its brand-name counterpart but is equally effective in
causing the desired response.

homocysteine: An amino acid (a substance used by the body to make proteins) that, when elevated in the blood, is believed to cause damage and
hardening of the arteries (atherosclerosis).

hormone: A substance released from a gland (such as the adrenal or thyroid gland) or cells in one part of the body that is transported in the blood and affects distant organs or cells. Examples include epinephrine, norepinephrine, and thyroxin.

hyperaldosteronism: An increase in the level of aldosterone, a hormone that is secreted from the adrenal gland and causes retention of sodium and water by the kidney; overproduction of aldosterone produces hypertension.

hyperlability: Marked instability; high changeability.

hyperthyroidism: Overactivity of the thyroid gland with increased secretion of thyroid hormones, which can result in a variety of characteristic signs and symptoms, including hypertension (usually systolic), prominent eyes, thyroid enlargement, excess sweating, weight loss, nervousness, and tremor.

hypertrophy: An enlargement or overgrowth of an organ or tissue.

hypotension: Abnormally low blood pressure that can cause lightheadedness, weakness, blurred vision, fainting, and unconsciousness.

hypothyroidism: Decreased activity of the thyroid gland accompanied by deficient release of thyroid hormone, which can result in a variety of signs and symptoms, sometimes including hypertension.

imaging: The production of images by radiologic, ultrasound, or magnetic resonance imaging (MRI) techniques.

imaging techniques: Techniques (such as CAT scan, MRI, X rays, ultrasound, and radioactive scans) that permit visualizing (seeing) areas of the body.

impedance to blood flow: Resistance to blood flow such as that occurring when vessels become constricted.

impotence: The inability to develop and/or sustain an erection and perform sexual intercourse.

intermittent claudication: Pain experienced in the lower extremities and sometimes in the hips and buttocks when walking due to diminished blood supply, usually caused by atherosclerosis.

ischemia: An inadequate blood supply to a part of the body.

labile hypertension: Blood pressure that may be normal sometimes and hypertensive at other times; fluctuations are especially pronounced.

LDL: See *low-density lipoprotein cholesterol.*

left ventricular hypertrophy (LVH): Enlargement of the muscle of the left (main) pumping chamber of the heart, which can result from hypertension because of the extra work required to pump blood effectively against elevated blood pressure.

libido: Sexual desire.

Liddle's syndrome: A genetic abnormality of the kidney, which retains sodium and excretes potassium in excessive amounts.

lipids: A general term for fats that includes the various types of cholesterol and the triglycerides.

lipoprotein: A combination of a lipid and protein.

low-density lipoprotein cholesterol (LDL): Also known as "bad" cholesterol. It can deposit cholesterol on the lining of blood vessels and cause obstructive plaques and atherosclerosis.

lupus: A chronic disease of unknown cause, which can cause changes in many tissues in the body, including the skin, lungs, kidneys, and joints.

LVH: See *left ventricular hypertrophy.*

magnesium: A mineral in the body that is required for many chemical reactions. A deficiency of magnesium causes irritability of the nervous system.

magnetic resonance imaging (MRI): An imaging technique employing magnetic energy rather than X rays.

manifestations: The signs and symptoms of a disease.

masked hypertension (reverse hypertension): A condition in which a patient exhibits normal blood pressure in a doctor's office but hypertension outside of the office.

metabolize: To biochemically build up or utilize substances to permit growth and energy in the body.

mm Hg: Millimeters (mm) of mercury (Hg); a volume of Hg is 13.5 times heavier than water. Blood pressure is expressed as mm Hg elevated in a glass tube recorded with a sphygmomanometer.

MRI: See *magnetic resonance imaging.*

multi-infarct dementia: A disorder that arises when multiple areas of the brain suffer damage caused by multiple strokes with impairment of brain function (e.g., memory and judgment deterioration, personality changes).

murmur: A blowing sound, often heard with a stethoscope over various areas of the heart (usually caused by abnormal heart valves) or over narrowed arteries. Sounds vary in quality and loudness and are the result of a disturbed blood flow.

myocardial infarction: An area of dead heart muscle caused by an impairment of the blood supply, usually due to blockage of a coronary artery.

neurohormone: A hormone used in the function of the nervous system. For example, norepinephrine is the neurohormone mainly responsible for the function of sympathetic nerves.

nitric oxide (NO): A substance released from the cells lining the arteries and arterioles, which causes relaxation of smooth muscle and dilation of the vessels.

NO: See *nitric oxide.*

nonsteroidal anti-inflammatory drugs (NSAIDs): NSAIDs include aspirin and aspirin-like drugs (Indacin, Motrin, Advil, Clinoril, Naprosyn). They block the enzyme responsible for the body's synthesis of prostaglandins and related substances. Blocking synthesis of some prostaglandins can cause salt and water retention by the kidney and thereby increase blood pressure.

norepinephrine (noradrenaline): A neurohormone released from sympathetic nerve endings and the adrenal gland, which can cause hypertension by constricting arteries and arterioles and can increase the rate and contraction of the heart.

NSAIDs: See *nonsteroidal anti-inflammatory drugs.*

ophthalmoscope: An instrument used to examine the interior of the eye.

osteoporosis: An abnormal decrease in bone density: namely, a thinning and loss of calcium and bone substance.

pallor: Paleness or a decrease in skin coloration in Caucasians.

palpable: Felt by touching.

papilledema: Swelling of the optic nerve that can be seen in the back of the eye with an opthalmoscope; it may occur when the blood pressure is severely elevated.

parathyroid glands: Four small glands situated in the neck beside the thyroid gland. These glands secrete parathyroid hormone, which is mainly concerned with calcium and phosphorous metabolism.

pheochromocytoma: A rare tumor that most frequently occurs in the adrenal gland but may occur elsewhere; it usually secretes epinephrine and norepinephrine, which cause many signs and symptoms, including hypertension.

pituitary gland: A small gland at the base of the brain that secretes substances that affect hormone production and bodily functions.

placebo: A "dummy," innocuous medical treatment used as a control when evaluating a drug or procedure. If the drug or procedure is effective, it should produce better results than a placebo.

platelets: Very small, cell-like structures in the circulation that are involved in blood clotting.

postural hypotension: An abnormal decrease in blood pressure that occurs upon standing and may be associated with lightheadedness, weakness, and fainting.

preeclampsia: A condition of unknown cause occurring in about 3 percent of individuals during the last three months of pregnancy, accompanied by hypertension, fluid retention, and proteinuria (protein in the urine).

primary hypertension: See *essential hypertension.*

prognosis: A forecast or predicted outcome of a disease; the prospects of recovery.

prostaglandins: A group of chemicals that are synthesized in the body.

Some can cause dilation of arterioles, whereas others can cause constriction and thereby affect blood pressure. Prostaglandins can also influence blood clotting. Their synthesis can be blocked by aspirin and other NSAIDs (nonsteroidal anti-inflammatory drugs).

pulse pressure: The difference between systolic and diastolic pressure (subtract the diastolic pressure from the systolic pressure).

receptor: A structure on a cell that can be stimulated by a specific hormone or chemical to cause a biological response.

renal: Related to the kidney.

renal artery stenosis: Narrowing of an artery to a kidney that, if severe, may cause hypertension by increasing renin. The renin then generates angiotensin, a powerful constrictor of arterioles.

renin: An enzyme that is released from the kidney into the circulation and generates angiotensin I (an inactive substance), which is then converted into angiotensin, a powerful constrictor of arteries and arterioles that can elevate blood pressure.

resistant hypertension: Hypertension that does not appear to respond to lifestyle changes and drug treatment.

risk factors (of hypertension): Factors that increase the risk of heart, brain, kidney, eye, and vascular damage (associated with hypertension).

secrete: Elaborate, give off, or produce.

sleep apnea: A periodic cessation of air flow through the mouth and nose during sleep.

sodium: A mineral that makes up 40 percent of sodium chloride, which is commonly used as table salt in cooking and in processed food. Some salt-sensitive people retain salt and water, which can cause hypertension.

sphygmomanometer: An instrument used for measuring arterial blood pressure.

stenosis: A narrowing or constriction.

stent: A metal device inserted into a blood vessel to keep blood flowing through the vessel.

stethoscope: An instrument used to listen to sounds made by the heart, the lungs, and arterial narrowing or pulsations (including sounds in the arm during blood pressure measurement).

stimulate: To excite and cause increased activity.

stress test: A type of test used to evaluate the effect of exercise on the electrical activity and function of the heart and on the blood flow in the coronary arteries.

stroke: Sudden brain injury due to inadequate blood supply, resulting from a blocked artery or hemorrhage due to a ruptured artery. Brain damage may be large or minimal following a small temporary blockage such as a TIA (transient ischemic attack, a "ministroke").

stroke-prone rats: Rats that have a greater tendency to develop stroke than other rats when they become hypertensive.

sympathetic nervous system: Part of the autonomic or "involuntary" nervous system over which we have no control. It consists of nerves that release norepinephrine, which constricts arteries and arterioles and increases the rate and force of heart contractions, thereby elevating blood pressure.

systole: A contraction of the heart, which pumps blood into the aorta.

systolic blood pressure: The pressure during systole, when the heart is contracting to pump blood into the aorta. It is the higher of the two numbers used to record blood pressure.

target organs: Organs that can be damaged by hypertension, especially arteries of the heart, brain, kidney, eye, and lower extremities.

therapeutic: Having a beneficial or curative effect.

therapy: Treatment.

thromboxane: A substance in the body that causes constriction of blood vessels and aggregation (clumping) of platelets.

thyroid gland: A gland located in the front of the neck that secretes thyroid hormones, which are important in body metabolism.

thyroid-stimulating hormone (TSH): A hormone released from the pituitary gland that stimulates thyroid function.

TIA: See *transient ischemic attack*.

transient ischemic attack (TIA): A temporary inadequate blood supply to an area of the brain that causes transient neurological manifestations, often due to a "ministroke" caused by a small blood clot.

triglycerides: Lipids (fats) in the blood that, if elevated, may contribute to atherosclerosis; severe elevations may also cause pancreatitis, which is an inflammation of the pancreas.

TSH: See *thyroid stimulating hormone*.

uremia: Excess accumulation of waste products and chemicals in the blood because of kidney failure and the inability to adequately excrete these substances in the urine.

vascular: Related to the vascular system, which is composed of blood vessels made up of large and small arteries, which are in turn connected by capillaries to small and large veins.

vasoconstrictor: A substance that constricts (i.e., narrows) blood vessels; constriction can be caused by substances normally present in the body and by some medications. Vasoconstriction of arterioles is mainly responsible for elevating blood pressure.

vasodilator: A substance that causes dilation (i.e., expansion) of blood vessels; dilation can be caused by substances normally present in the body and by some medications. The dilation of arterioles is mainly responsible for lowering blood pressure.

veins: Blood vessels that return blood from the body and the lungs to the heart. Blood returning from the body requires replenishing of its oxygen content, which was removed by the tissues. Blood is oxygenated in the lungs and then returned to the left ventricle, which pumps it into the aorta.

ventricle: The two large pumping chambers of the heart. The right ventricle pumps blood to the lungs, whereas the left ventricle, which has a muscle wall three times thicker than that of the right ventricle, pumps blood to all parts of the body.

vitamin: A general term for substances that occur in many plant and animal foods and are necessary in extremely small amounts for normal body function.

white-coat hypertension: Hypertension that occurs in the doctor's office but does not occur at home or elsewhere. Anxiety and fear in the doctor's office are probably responsible for this type of temporary hypertension.

— Index —

Figures and tables are indicated with *f* and *t*, respectively.

— About the Authors ————————————

Ray W. Gifford, Jr., MD
The late Ray W. Gifford, Jr., MD (1923–2004), was
past president of the National Hypertension Association and past chairman, Department of Nephrology
and Hypertension at the Cleveland Clinic. He served
as chairman of the *Fifth Joint National Committee on
Prevention, Detection, Evaluation, and Treatment of
High Blood Pressure (JNC V)* in 1991–1992. He had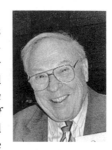
also been a member of the Coordinating Committee
of the National High Blood Pressure Education Program of the National
Heart, Lung, and Blood Institute since 1980. Dr. Gifford was the author of
over 450 scientific papers and served on the editorial boards of many jour-
nals including the *Journal of Cardiovascular Risk, Hypertension Research —
Clinical and Experimental, Stroke,* and the *American Journal of Cardiology.*
He was the recipient of numerous awards including the Lifetime Achievement Award in Hypertension from the Council on High Blood Pressure
Research of the American Heart Association. In 1993 the Ray W. Gifford,
Jr., MD, endowed chair in hypertension was established at the Cleveland
Clinic Foundation. In 1997 he was inducted into the Medical Hall of Fame
of Cleveland, Ohio.

William M. Manger, MD, PhD, FACP, FACC
Dr. Manger received his bachelor of science degree
from Yale University in 1944 and his medical degree
from Columbia College of Physicians and Surgeons in
1946. Between 1950–1955 he was a Fellow in Medicine
at the Mayo Clinic and obtained a PhD from the Uni-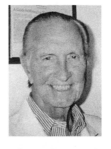
versity of Minnesota in 1958. He received the Mayo
Foundation Alumni Award for Meritorious Research
in 1955 for his work on the quantitation of epineph-
rine and norepinephrine in plasma. Since 1958 he has performed research
in areas including hemorrhagic shock, hypertension, sympatho-adrenal
responses, pheochromocytoma, the mechanism of salt-induced hypertension, and the growth of tumor cells.
    Dr. Manger has served in the Department of Medicine as professor of
clinical medicine at New York University Medical Center since 1983. He is
a lecturer in medicine (emeritus) at Columbia Medical School. In 1992 he
was designated Distinguished Mayo Foundation Alumnus in recognition

of his exceptional national and international research, medical practice, and education in hypertension. In 2009 he was awarded the Mayo Clinic Alumni Association Humanitarian Award for his exceptional contributions, dedication, and achievements in improving public health, particularly as a true pioneer in the prevention of childhood obesity, one of the single greatest threats to health in this country.

Dr. Manger has a lifelong history of emphasizing the civic message of prevention as the first course of action with chronic illnesses. Over his career, he has written and co-authored five medical books and more than 240 scientific publications. In 1977 he founded the National Hypertension Association (NHA), gradually building up an impressive board of trustees and contributors. Under his leadership, the NHA has conducted groundbreaking research on hypertension. Seven years ago, when obesity in children came to the forefront, he and his wife established VITAL (Value Initiative Teaching About Lifestyle) as a humanitarian health measure. The primary purpose of *VITAL* is to educate children — from preschool to third grade — in the prevention of unhealthy lifestyles.

Throughout his career as basic researcher and tertiary-care clinician, Dr. Manger has chosen to devote his time, resources, and unbridled energy to improve lives — especially of the underserved and those yet to be served — which are the reasons the Mayo brothers established the Mayo Clinic.

Norman M. Kaplan, MD, MACP

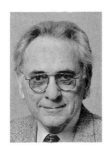

Dr. Kaplan is clinical professor of internal medicine at the University of Texas Southwestern Medical Center at Dallas where he has been on the faculty for more than forty years. For the last twenty years his teaching, writing, and research have focused primarily upon clinical aspects of hypertension. He has lectured extensively and contributed over five hundred papers to the medical literature. The tenth edition of his textbook, *Kaplan's Clinical Hypertension*, was published in 2009. He was a member of the third, fourth, fifth, and sixth Joint National Committee on Prevention, Detection, Evaluation, and Treatment of High Blood Pressure. He has been made a Master of the American College of Physicians, given the Lifetime Achievement Award by the American Heart Association's Council for High Blood Pressure Research, and received the Stevo Julius Award for Leadership in Medical Communication presented by the International Society of Hypertension. He served on the executive committees of the American Society of Hypertension and the AHA Council for High Blood Pressure Research. He is involved as either editor or reviewer with most of the journals that publish papers in the hypertension arena.

Edward J. Roccella, PhD, MPH

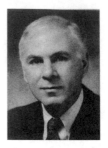

Edward Roccella received his bachelor of science degree from East Tennessee State University. He continued his education at the University of Michigan and earned a master of public health and doctor of philosophy degree in health education and health behavior. Dr. Roccella began his professional career as director of continuing education at the University of Pittsburgh Regional Medical Program and as an instructor in community medicine. Subsequently, he became an assistant professor at the University of Michigan Medical School and School of Public Health. In 1978 he began work at the National Institutes of Health in Bethesda, Maryland, as coordinator of the National High Blood Pressure Education Program (NHBPEP). In this position he directed the NHBPEP public, patient, and professional activities, which have been cited to improve the nation's hypertension profile, and contributed to the nation's large decline in cardiovascular disease. As NHBPEP coordinator he organized forty-five professional, voluntary, and official organizations into one body that developed national clinical guidelines for the prevention and treatment of hypertension. The NHBPEP issues several reports, one of which is the Joint National Committee report. He has led United States scientific exchange delegations regarding the prevention and treatment of hypertension to Brazil, Germany, Egypt, and Jordan.

Dr. Roccella has authored 107 publications in scientific journals and textbooks dealing with the prevention and control of high blood pressure, patient education, public health approaches to improving cardiovascular health, and evaluating large-scale public health programs. He is a past president of the Society for Public Health Education and a former member of the American Public Health Association Governing Council, and he serves as a referee for several national and international scientific and medical journals.

Dr. Roccella has been awarded the National Institutes of Health Directors Award, the HealthTrac Foundation Prize, the University of Michigan John Romani Prize for lifetime achievement in public health administration, the American Society of Hypertension Presidents Award, the International Society of Hypertension in Blacks Presidential Award, the Society for Public Health Education Distinguished Fellow, and the 2008 Senator Frank Laughtenberg Award. He retired from the National Institutes of Health in 2007 but remains active in the field of cardiovascular disease prevention and control and serves on the medical/public health advisory boards of four national professional and advocacy organizations.